Study Guide for

Nursing Research: Methods and Critical Appraisal for Evidence-Based Practice

8th Edition

Geri LoBiondo-Wood, PhD, RN, FAAN
Professor and Coordinator, PhD in Nursing Program
University of Texas Health Science Center at Houston
School of Nursing
Houston, Texas

Judith Haber, PhD, APRN, BC, FAAN
The Ursula Springer Leadership Professor in Nursing
Associate Dean for Graduate Programs
New York University
College of Nursing
New York, New York

Study Guide prepared by:

Carey A. Berry, MS, BSN, RN
Formerly, Clinical Nurse
Gastrointestinal Surgical Oncology
M.D. Anderson Cancer Center
The University of Texas
Denver, Colorado

Jennifer Yost, PhD, RN
Assistant Professor
School of Nursing, Faculty of Health Sciences
McMaster University
Hamilton, Ontario
Canada

ELSEVIER
MOSBY

ELSEVIER

MOSBY

3251 Riverport Lane
St. Louis, Missouri 63043

Study Guide for Nursing Research: Methods and Critical Appraisal for
Evidence-Based Practice, Eighth Edition

978-0-323-22643-1

Notices

Knowledge and best practice in this field are constantly changing. As new research and experience broaden our knowledge, changes in practice, treatment and drug therapy may become necessary or appropriate. Readers are advised to check the most current information provided (i) on procedures featured or (ii) by the manufacturer of each product to be administered, to verify the recommended dose or formula, the method and duration of administration, and contraindications. It is the responsibility of the practitioner, relying on their own experience and knowledge of the patient, to make diagnoses, to determine dosages and the best treatment for each individual patient, and to take all appropriate safety precautions. To the fullest extent of the law, neither the Publisher nor the authors assume any liability for any injury and/or damage to persons or property arising out of or related to any use of the material contained in this book.

International Standard Book Number: 978-0-323-22643-1

Executive Content Strategist: Lee Henderson
Content Manager: Jennifer Ehlers
Content Coordinator: Courtney Daniels
Publishing Services Manager: Jeffrey Patterson
Senior Project Manager: Anne Konopka

Printed in the United States of America

Last digit is the print number: 9 8 7 6 5 4 3 2

Introduction

Information bombards us! The student lament used to be, "I can't find any information on X." Now the cry is, "What do I do with all of the information on X?" The focus shifts from finding information to thinking about how to use and filter information. What information is worth keeping? What should be discarded? What is useful to clinical practice? What is fluff? Where are the gaps?

Thinking about the links between information and practice is critical to the improvement of the nursing care we deliver. As each of us strengthens our individual understanding of the links between interventions and outcomes, we move nursing's collective practice closer to being truly evidence-based. We can "know" what intervention works best in what situation.

"Helping people get better safely and efficiently" begins with thinking. Our intent is that the activities in the Study Guide will help you strengthen your skills in thinking about information found in the literature. The activities are designed to assist you in evaluating the research you read so you are prepared to undertake the critical analysis of research studies. As you practice the appraisal skills addressed in this Study Guide, you will be strengthening your ability to make evidence-based practice decisions grounded in theory and research.

What an incredible time to be a nurse!

GENERAL DIRECTIONS

1. We recommend that you read the textbook chapter first, then complete the Study Guide activities for that chapter.

2. Complete each Study Guide chapter in order. The Study Guide is designed so that you build on the knowledge gained in Chapter 1 to complete the activities in Chapter 2, and so forth. The activities are designed to give you the opportunity to apply the knowledge learned in the textbook and actually use this knowledge to solve problems, thereby gaining increased confidence that comes only from working through each chapter.

3. Follow the specific directions that precede each activity. Be certain that you have the resources needed to complete the activity before you begin.

4. Take the posttest in each Study Guide chapter after you have completed all of the chapter's activities. The answers for the posttest items can be found in the answer key. If you answer 85% of the questions correctly, be confident that you have grasped the essential material presented in the chapter.

5. Clarify any questions, confusion, or concerns you may have with your instructor.

ACTIVITY ANSWERS ARE IN THE BACK OF THIS BOOK

Answers in a workbook such as this do not follow a formula like answers in a math book. Many times you are asked to make a judgment about a particular problem. If your judgment differs from that of the authors, review the criteria that you used to make your decision. Determine if you followed a logical progression of steps to reach your conclusion. If not, rework the activity. If the process you followed appears logical, and your answer remains different, remember that even experts may disagree on many of the judgment calls in nursing research. There will continue to be many "gray areas." If you average an 85% agreement with the authors, you can be sure that you are on the right track and should feel very confident about your level of expertise.

Carey A. Berry, MS, BSN, RN

Jennifer Yost, PhD, RN

Contents

PART IV   APPLICATION OF RESEARCH: EVIDENCE-BASED PRACTICE

Integrating Research, Evidence-Based Practice, and Quality Improvement Processes

INTRODUCTION

One goal of this chapter is to assist you in reviewing the material presented in Chapter 1 of the text written by LoBiondo-Wood and Haber. A second and more fundamental goal is to provide you with an opportunity to begin practicing the role of a critical consumer of research. Succeeding chapters in this study guide fine-tune your ability to evaluate research studies critically.

LEARNING OUTCOMES

On completion of this chapter, you should be able to do the following:

- State the significance of research to evidence-based nursing practice.
- Identify the role of the consumer of nursing research.
- Define *evidence-based practice.*
- Discuss evidence-based decision making.
- Explain the difference between quantitative and qualitative research.
- Explain the difference among types of systematic reviews: integrative review, meta-analysis, and meta-synthesis.
- Identify the importance of critical thinking and critical reading skills for critical appraisal of research studies.
- Discuss the format and style of research reports/articles.
- Discuss how to use a quantitative evidence hierarchy when critically appraising research studies.

Activity 1

Match the term in Column B with the appropriate phrase in Column A. Each term will be used only once. This may be a good time to review the glossary and the key terms in Chapter 1.

Column A

Column B

1. __C__   Systematic investigation about phenomena   C

2. __d__   Studies conducted to understand the meaning   b of human experience

3. __b__   Statistical technique used to summarize studies   a in a systematic review

4. __a__   Critically evaluates a research report's content based on a set of criteria to evaluate the   e scientific merit for application to practice

5. __g__   Studies conducted to test relationships, assess differences, and/or explain cause and effect

6. __e__   Summary and assessment of a group that considered similar research questions

7. __f__   Clinical practice based on the collection, evaluation, and integration of clinical expertise,   f research evidence, and patient preferences

8. __h__   Systematically developed statements that provide recommendations to guide practice   h

9. __i__   Systematic use of data to monitor outcomes of   i care

Column B

a. Critique
b. Meta-analysis (many analyses)
c. Research
d. Qualitative
e. Systematic review
f. Evidence-based practice
g. Quantitative
h. Clinical guidelines
i. Quality improvement

Activity 2

Match the term in Column B with the appropriate phrase in Column A. Terms from Column B will be used more than once.

Column A

Column B

1. __b__   Getting a general sense of the material

2. __b__   Clarifying unfamiliar terms with text

3. __a__   Using constructive skepticism

4. __a__   Questioning assumptions

5. __a__   Rationally examining ideas

6. __a__   Thinking about your own thinking

7. __b__   Allowing assessment of study validity

a. Critical thinking
b. Critical reading

Activity 3

Complete each item with the appropriate word or phrase from the text.

1. Key variables, new terms, and steps of the research process should be identified following a(n) _____ understanding of a research article.

2. With _____ understanding of a research article, you should be able to state the main purpose of the study in one or two sentences.

3. Analysis of an article will allow understanding of the _____ of a study; synthesis will allow understanding of the _____ article and all steps in the research process.

Activity 4: Evidence-Based Practice Activity

1. For Appendix B (Alhusen et al., 2012), Appendix D (Melvin et al., 2012), and Appendix E (Murphy et al., 2012), identify the articles' level of evidence using Figure 1-1 in your textbook.

   a. Melvin et al., 2012: _____

   b. Alhusen et al., 2012: _____

   c. Murphy et al., 2012: _____

2. Find a research article in your area of practice and determine the level of evidence for the article.

Activity 5

Match the term in Column B with the appropriate phrase in Column A.

	Column A	**Column B**
1. _____	Extent to which a study's design, implementation, and analysis minimize bias	a. Consistency b. Quality c. Quantity
2. _____	Degree to which studies that have similar and different designs, but consider the same research question, report similar findings	
3. _____	Number of studies that have evaluated the research question, as well as the strength of the findings from the data analyses	

Activity 6

Using Appendix A (Thomas et al., 2012), determine where in the article the following steps of the research process are identified:

1. Research problem:_____

2. Purpose: _____

3. Literature review: _____

4. Theoretical framework and/or conceptual framework:_____

5. Hypothesis/research questions:_____

6. Research design: _____

7. Sample—type and size: _____

8. Legal-ethical issues:_____

9. Instruments: _____

10. Validity and reliability: _____

11. Data collection procedure: _____

12. Data analysis:_____

13. Results: _____

14. Discussion of findings and new findings: _____

15. Implications, limitations, and recommendations:_____

POSTTEST

1. To read a research study critically, the reader must have skilled reading, writing, and reasoning abilities. Use these abilities to read the following abstract, and then identify concepts, clarify any unfamiliar concepts or terms, and question any assumptions or rationales presented.

    In this study we examined pain and disability in 115 community-dwelling, urban, older adults. . . . Sixty percent of the sample reported experiencing pain. In this sample, 66 (57.4%) participants reported having physical limitations in at least one item on the physical mobility subscale of the SIP. Pain is a common problem, and its high prevalence (60%) in this sample of individuals over 60 years of age is consistent with epidemiological studies of pain. . . . Pain was significantly associated with greater functional disability in both physical and social functional domains, highlighting the important real-world consequences of living with pain. Contrary to previous research, race was not related to pain in this sample (Horgas et al., 2008).

    a.   Identify the concepts.

    b.   List any unfamiliar concepts or terms that you would need to clarify.

    c.   What assumptions or rationales would you question?

2.   Identify one <u>similarity</u> between research and evidence-based practice.

3.   Identify one <u>difference</u> between research and evidence-based practice.

4.   Identify one <u>similarity</u> between quantitative and qualitative research.

5.   Identify one <u>difference</u> between quantitative and qualitative research.

REFERENCES

Alhusen, J. L., Gross, D., Hayat, M. J., et al. (2012). The influence of maternal-fetal attachment and health practices on neonatal outcome in low-income, urban women. *Research in Nursing & Health, 35,* 112-120.

Horgas A. L., Yoon S. L., Nichols A. L., et al. (2008). The relationship between pain and functional disability in black and white older adults. *Research in Nursing & Health, 31*(4), 341-354.

Melvin, K. C., Gross, D., Hayat, M. J., et al. (2012). Couple functioning and post-traumatic stress symptoms in US Army couples: The role of resilience. *Research in Nursing & Health, 35,* 164-177.

Murphy, F. A., Lipp, A., & Powles, D. L. (2012). Follow-up for improving psychological well being for women after a miscarriage. *Cochrane Database of Systematic Reviews, 3,* CD008679. DOI: 10.1002/14651858.CD008679.pub2.

Thomas, M. L., Elliot, J. E., Rao, S. M., et al. (2012). A randomized, clinical trial of education or motivational-interviewing-based coaching compared to usual care to improve cancer pain management. *Oncology Nursing Forum, 39*(1), 39-49.

Research Questions, Hypotheses, and Clinical Questions

INTRODUCTION

This chapter focuses on identifying research questions, hypotheses, and clinical questions. If developed correctly, research questions can be very helpful to you as a research consumer because they concisely describe the essence of the research study. Research questions present the idea that is to be examined in the study. Hypotheses, which extend from the literature review and research questions, are predictions that provide a vehicle for testing the relationships between variables. For the nurse who considers using the results of a given study in practice, the two primary concerns are to locate and critique the research question and the hypotheses. The research question or hypotheses provide the most succinct link between the underlying theoretical base and guide the design of the research study. Although similar to research questions, clinical questions are developed by the nurse to provide answers to clinical situations. Clinical questions, framed using the PICO (population, intervention, comparison, outcome) format, are the basis for searching the literature to identify the best available evidence for clinical situations.

LEARNING OUTCOMES

On completion of this chapter, you should be able to do the following:

- Describe how the research question and hypothesis relate to the other components of the research process.
- Describe the process of identifying and refining a research question or hypothesis.
- Identify the criteria for determining the significance of a research question or hypothesis.
- Discuss the purpose of developing a clinical question.
- Discuss the appropriate use of the purpose, aim, or objective of a research study.
- Discuss how the purpose, research question, and hypothesis suggest the level of evidence to be obtained from the findings of a research study.
- Discuss the appropriate use of research questions versus hypotheses in a research study.
- Discuss the differences between a research question and a clinical question in relation to evidence-based practice.
- Apply the critiquing criteria to the evaluation of a research question and hypothesis in a research report.

Activity 1

Match the terms in Column B to the appropriate phrase in Column A.

Column A

1. __f__ Statement about the relationship among two or more variables
2. __b__ Variable that has the presumed effect on another variable
3. __d__ Nonmanipulated variable that the researcher is interested in understanding, explaining, or predicting
4. __a__ Property of the research question that variables must lend themselves to observation, measurement, and analysis
5. __c__ Concepts or properties that are operationalized and studied
6. __e__ Statement that presents the idea(s) to be examined in the study

Column B

a. Testability
b. Independent variable
c. Variables
d. Dependent variable
e. Research question
f. Hypothesis

Activity 2

A good research question exhibits three characteristics. Critique the research questions below to determine if each of the three criteria is present. Following each problem statement is a list representing the three criteria (a, b, and c). Circle *yes* or *no* to indicate whether each criterion is met.

The research question:

a. Clearly identifies the variable(s) under consideration
b. Specifies the population being studied
c. Implies the possibility of empirical testing

1. The purpose of this study was to compare substance involvement among adolescent smokers in a psychiatric inpatient facility who had received either a motivational interviewing intervention or brief advice for smoking cessation (Brown et al., 2009).
   Criterion a: (Yes) No
   Criterion b: (Yes) No
   Criterion c: (Yes) No

2. The purpose of this study was to determine if a predictive relationship exists between critical thinking and success in nursing. Success in nursing was defined as passing the NCLEX-RN® on the first attempt (Shirrell, 2008).
   Criterion a: (Yes) No
   Criterion b: (Yes) No
   Criterion c: Yes (No)

3. The purpose of this study was to describe the experience of the use of community services, including benefits and barriers, by family caregivers of relatives with Alzheimer's disease or a related disorder (Winslow, 2003).

   Criterion a: Yes   No
   Criterion b: Yes   No
   Criterion c: Yes   No

4. The purpose of this study was to assess self-perception of body weight among a selected sample of Taipei, Taiwan, high school students and other weight-related factors such as weight management practices, weight management goal, weight satisfaction, perception of physical attractiveness, and normative perceptions of schoolmates regarding weight loss (Page et al., 2005).

   Criterion a: Yes   No
   Criterion b: Yes   No
   Criterion c: Yes   No

5. The aim of this study was to explore cancer patients' experiences of nursing pain management during hospitalization for cancer treatment (Rustøen et al., 2009).

   Criterion a: Yes   No
   Criterion b: Yes   No
   Criterion c: Yes   No

Activity 3

Research questions are used to guide all types of research studies. Identify whether you would expect a quantitative or qualitative research study design from the research questions in Activity 2.

Key:
   a. Quantitative
   b. Qualitative

1. A   The purpose of this study was to compare substance involvement among adolescent smokers in a psychiatric inpatient facility who had received either a motivational interviewing intervention or brief advice for smoking cessation (Brown et al., 2009).

2. A   The purpose of this study was to determine if a predictive relationship exists between critical thinking and success in nursing. Success in nursing was defined as passing the NCLEX-RN® on the first attempt (Shirrell, 2008).

3.  B   The purpose of this study was to describe the experience of the use of community services, including benefits and barriers, by family caregivers of relatives with Alzheimer's disease or a related disorder (Winslow, 2003).

4. A   The purpose of this study was to assess self-perception of body weight among a selected sample of Taipei, Taiwan, high school students and other weight-related factors such as weight management practices, weight management goal, weight satisfaction, perception of physical attractiveness, and normative perceptions of schoolmates regarding weight loss (Page et al., 2005).

5.  B   The aim of this study was to explore cancer patients' experiences of nursing pain management during hospitalization for cancer treatment (Rustøen et al., 2009).

Activity 4

The ability to distinguish between independent and dependent variables is crucial in critiquing a research hypothesis to determine whether it is a succinct statement of the relationship between two variables. Determine the independent variable and the dependent variable in each of the following research hypotheses.

1. Regular provision of iron improves iron status of breast-fed infants without adverse effects (Zeigler et al., 2009).

    a. Independent variable:

    b. Dependent variable:

2. Family-centered care is a significant predictor of children's health-related quality of life, independent of illness severity (Moore et al., 2009).

    a. Independent variable:

    b. Dependent variable:

3. There is no difference between continuous nebulization of albuterol at 7.5 mg/hr (usual dose) and 15 mg/hr (high dose) in peak flow improvement up to 3 hours in patients with acute bronchospasm (Stein & Levitt, 2003).

    a. Independent variable:

    b. Dependent variable:

4. People who report more frequent or more recent dental prophylaxes are more likely to have better glycemic control (Taylor et al., 2005).

    a. Independent variable:

    b. Dependent variable:

5. More supportive/less negative parenting is associated with lower resting blood pressure and heart rates in children (Bell & Belsky, 2008).

    a. Independent variable:

    b. Dependent variable:

Activity 5

Take each hypothesis from Activity 4 and label it with the appropriate abbreviation from the key provided.

Key: DH = Directional hypothesis
NDH = Nondirectional hypothesis

1. _____ Regular provision of iron improves iron status of breast-fed infants without adverse effects (Ziegler et al., 2009).

2. _____ Family-centered care is a significant predictor of children's health-related quality of life, independent of illness severity (Moore et al., 2009).

3. _____ There is no difference between continuous nebulization of albuterol at 7.5 mg/hr (usual dose) and 15 mg/hr (high dose) in peak flow improvement up to 3 hours in the patients with acute bronchospasm (Stein & Levitt, 2003).

4. _____ People who report more frequent or more recent dental prophylaxes are more likely to have better glycemic control (Taylor et al., 2005).

5. _____ More supportive/less negative parenting is associated with lower resting blood pressure and heart rates in children (Bell & Belsky, 2008).

Activity 6

Critique the following hypothesis.

African-American women with higher levels of depression will have higher blood pressure levels, more cardiovascular risk factors, greater stress, and lower social support (Artinian et al., 2006).

1. Is the hypothesis clearly stated in a declarative form?

    Yes   No

2. Are the independent and dependent variables identified in the statement of the hypothesis?

    Yes   No

3. Are the variables measurable or potentially measurable?

    Yes   No

4. Is the hypothesis stated in such a way that it is testable?

    Yes   No

5. Is the hypothesis stated objectively without value-laden words?

    Yes   No

6. Is the direction of the relationship in the hypothesis clearly stated?

    Yes   No

7. Is each of the hypotheses specific to one relationship so that each hypothesis can be either supported or not supported?

    Yes   No

Activity 7

Clinical questions often arise from clinical situations. Using the PICO format for formulating clinical questions helps practicing nurses identify the best available evidence on which to base clinical and health care decisions. In the following clinical questions, identify the four components of clinical questions.

1. In children presenting to the emergency department with acute long-bone fractures, is intranasal fentanyl equivalent to intravenous morphine for pain control? (Yost, 2007)

    P: _____

    I: _____

    C: _____

    O: _____

2. Is a group intervention for parents and children more effective than routine care for weight loss in obese school-age children? (Heale, 2008)

    P: _____

    I: _____

    C: _____

    O: _____

3. What are the experiences of men after laparoscopic radical prostatectomy? (Mick, 2009)

    P: _____

    I: _____

    C: _____

    O: _____

POSTTEST

Refer to the article by Thomas et al. (2012) in Appendix A of your textbook.

1. Highlight the research question.

2. Does the research question indicate a quantitative or qualitative research design?

3. Critique the research question by answering yes or no to the following questions. Does the research question:

   a. Clearly identify the variable(s) under consideration?

   b. Specify the population being studied?

   c. Imply the possibility of empirical testing?

4. Put the research question into the PICO format for clinical questions.

5. List the variables being studied. Identify the independent variable(s) and dependent variable(s).

6. Is there a hypothesis stated by the researchers? If yes, highlight the hypothesis. Is the hypothesis directional or nondirectional?

REFERENCES

Artinian, N. T., Washington, O. G. M., Flack, J. M., et al. (2006). Depression, stress, and blood pressure in urban African-American women. *Progress in Cardiovascular Nursing, 21*(2), 68-75.

Bell, B. G., & Belsky, J. (2008). Parenting and children's cardiovascular functioning. *Child: Care, Health, and Development, 34*(2), 194-203.

Brown, R. A., Strong, D. R., Abrantes, A. M., et al. (2009). Effects on substance use outcomes in adolescents receiving motivational interviewing for smoking cessation during psychiatric hospitalization. *Addictive Behaviors, 34*(10), 887-891.

Heale, R. (2008). A group intervention for parents and children achieved greater weight loss in obese children than routine care. *Evidence-Based Nursing, 11*, 43.

Mick, J. (2009). Men were surprised by the severity of symptoms they experienced after laparoscopic radical prostatectomy. *Evidence-Based Nursing, 12*, 28.

Page, R. M., Lee, C., Miao, N. (2005). Self perception of body weight among high school students in Taipei, Taiwan. *International Journal of Adolescent Medicine and Health, 17*(2), 123-136.

Rustøen, T., Gaardsrud, M., Leegaard, M., & Wahl, A. K. (2009). Nursing pain management: A qualitative interview study of patients with pain, hospitalized for cancer treatment. *Pain Management Nursing, 10*(1), 48-55.

Shirrell, D. (2008). Critical thinking as a predictor of success in an associate degree nursing program. *Teaching and Learning in Nursing, 3*(4), 131-136.

Stein, J., & Levitt, M. A. (2003). A randomized, controlled double-blind trial of usual-dose versus high-dose albuterol via continuous nebulization in patients with acute bronchospasm. *Annals of Emergency Medicine, 10*(1), 31-36.

Taylor, G. W., Pritzel, S. J., Manz, M. C., Borgnakke, W. S., Eber, R. M., & Bouman, P. D. (2005). Frequency of dental prophylaxis and glycemic control in type 2 diabetes. *Journal of Dental Hygiene, 79*(4), 22-25. Retrieved from http://www.ingentaconnect.com/content/adha/jdh;jsessionid=7hnhm8si722gp.alice.

Thomas, M. L., Elliott, J. E., Rao, S. M., et al. (2012). A randomized clinical trial of education or motivational interviewing based coaching compared to usual care to improve cancer pain management. *Oncology Nursing Forum, 39*(1), 39-49.

Winslow, B. W. (2003). Family caregivers' experiences with community services: A qualitative analysis. *Public Health Nursing, 20*(5), 341-348.

Yost, J. (2007). Intranasal fentanyl and intravenous morphine did not differ for pain relief in children with closed long-bone fractures. *Evidence-Based Nursing, 11*, 42.

Ziegler, E. E., Nelson, S. E., & Jeter, J. M. (2009). Iron status of breastfed infants is improved equally by medicinal iron and iron-fortified cereal. *American Journal of Clinical Nutrition, 90*(1), 76-87.

Gathering and Appraising the Literature

INTRODUCTION

The phrases *literature review* or *review of the literature* refer to a key step in the research process for researchers, as well as for consumers of research. For researchers, the *literature review* is the section of a research study in which the researcher retrieves, critically appraises, and synthesizes previously existing knowledge. It is this literature review that is then used as the basis for the development of research questions and hypotheses by the researcher. Similarly, as consumers of research, nurses involved in evidence-based practice are also responsible for *reviewing the literature*. They systematically gather, critically appraise, and synthesize the best-available evidence to establish its strength, quality, and consistency to determine its applicability to practice. This chapter will help you learn more about how to critique the literature review performed by researchers and how to conduct a literature review as a consumer of research to address clinical questions.

LEARNING OUTCOMES

On completion of this chapter, you should be able to do the following:

- Discuss the relationship of the literature review to nursing theory, research, education, and practice.
- Differentiate the purposes of the literature review from the perspective of the research investigator and the research consumer.
- Discuss the use of the literature review for quantitative designs and qualitative methods.
- Discuss the purpose of reviewing the literature in developing evidence-based practice and quality improvement projects.
- Differentiate between primary and secondary sources.
- Compare the advantages and disadvantages of the most commonly used online databases and print database sources for conducting a literature review.
- Identify the characteristics of an effective electronic search of the literature.
- Critically read, appraise, and synthesize primary and secondary sources used for the development of a literature review.
- Apply critiquing criteria to the evaluation of literature reviews in selected research studies.

Activity 1

Sometimes it is difficult to understand the distinction between primary and secondary sources of information. A comparison that is always helpful is if you are considering giving a patient an injection for pain, whose report would you feel most comfortable evaluating—the report of a family member or nurse's aide (i.e., secondary source) or the report by the patient (i.e., primary source)? As a consumer of nursing research, you will also need to evaluate the credibility of literature in part on whether it is generated from primary or secondary sources so that you know whether you are reading a first-hand report or someone else's interpretation of the material. Below is a selected list of references from the study by Melvin et al. (2012) (Appendix D in the textbook). Next to each reference, indicate whether it is a primary (*P*) or secondary (*S*) source. Sometimes it is helpful to retrieve the abstract or full text of the reference.

1. __P__ Blake, D. D., Weathers, F. W., Nagy, L. M., et al. (1995). The development of a clinician-administered PTSD scale. *Journal of Traumatic Stress, 8*, 75-90.

2. __S__ Dekel, R., & Solomon, Z. (2007). Secondary traumatization among wives of war veterans with PTSD. In C. Figley & W. Nash (Eds.). *Combat stress injury: Theory, research, and management.* London: Routledge.

3. __S__ Figley, C. R. (1995). Compassion fatigue as secondary traumatic stress disorder: An overview. In C. R. Figley (Ed.). *Compassion fatigue* (pp. 1-20). New York, NY: Brunner/Mazel.

4. __P__ Houry, D., Rhodes, K. V., Kemball, R. S., et al. (2008). Differences in female and male victims and perpetrators of partner violence with respect to WEB scores. *Journal of Interpersonal Violence, 23*, 1041-1055. DOI: 10.1177/0886260507313969.

Activity 2

Typically a literature review consists of numerous journal articles. Whether the review of literature is being conducted by a researcher or a consumer of research, attempts should be made to retrieve articles from refereed or peer-reviewed journals. Below is a selected list of references from the study by Melvin et al. (2012) (Appendix D in the textbook). Next to each reference, indicate whether it is a peer-reviewed journal (*PR*) or non–peer-reviewed journal (*NPR*). Note: It may be helpful to look up the journal online.

1. _____ Busby, D. M., Christensen, C., Crane, D. R., & Larson, J. H. (1995). A revision of the Dyadic Adjustment Scale for use with distressed and nondistressed couples: Construct hierarchy and multidimensional scales. *Journal of Marital and Family Therapy, 21*, 289-308.

2. _____ Campbell, J. C., Garza, M. A., Gielen, A. C., et al. (2003). Intimate partner violence and abuse among active duty military women. *Violence Against Women, 9*, 1072-1092.

3. _____ Coker, A. L., Pope, B. O., Smith, P. H., et al. (2001). Assessment of clinical partner violence screening tools. *Journal of American Medical Women's Association, 56*, 19-23.

4. _____ Connor, K. M., & Davidson, J. R. T. (2003). Development of a new resilience scale: The Connor–Davidson Resilience Scale (CD-RISC). *Depression and Anxiety, 18*, 76-82.

5. _____ Elhai, J. D., Gray, M. J., Docherty, A. R., et al. (2007). Structural validity of the Posttraumatic Stress Disorder Checklist among college students with a trauma history. *Journal of Interpersonal Violence, 22,* 1471-1478.

6. _____ Hoge, C. W., Auchertonie, J. L., & Milliken, C. S. (2006). Mental health problems, use of mental health services, and attrition from military service after returning from deployment to Iraq or Afghanistan. *Journal of the American Medical Association, 295,* 1023-1032.

Activity 3: Web-Based Activity

Although there are books, journals, and additional literature that remain only available in print versions located in libraries, the Internet has become a major source for researchers and consumers of research conducting reviews of the literature. Two of the most common Internet sources are (1) online bibliographic and abstract databases and (2) online search engines. Conduct a basic search of CINAHL (the most relevant and frequently used source for nursing literature) and Google (an online search engine) using the following search terms: "postmenopausal women" and "exercise" and "osteoporosis." Compare the literature retrieved.

1. How many items were retrieved from CINAHL?

2. How many items were retrieved from Google?

3. Which source retrieved the most relevant, peer-reviewed journal articles?

4. Which source would be the best use of your time for gathering literature in a scholarly way?

Activity 4: Web-Based Activity

Retrieve and review the following articles:

Haynes, R. B. (2001). Of studies, syntheses, synopses, and systems: The "4S" evolution of services for finding current best evidence. *Evidence-Based Medicine, 6,* 36-38.
Haynes, R. B. (2007). Of studies, summaries, synopses, summaries and systems: The "5S" evolution of information services for evidence-based healthcare decisions. *Evidence-Based Nursing, 10,* 6-7.
DiCenso, A., Bayley, L., & Haynes, B. (2009). Accessing pre-appraised evidence: Fine tuning the 5S model into a 6S model. *Evidence-Based Nursing, 12*(4), 99-101.

1. Describe how the 6S Pyramid has evolved over time from the 4S Pyramid. What levels of the pyramid have not changed over time? What levels have been added over time?

Activity 5

The review of the literature is usually easy to find. In the abridged version of a research study, it is most frequently labeled *Review of Literature* or *Relevant Literature* or something comparable. It may also be separated into a literature review section and another section titled *Conceptual Framework* that presents material on the theoretical or conceptual framework. Critically appraising the literature review of research studies is a necessary step for both researchers and consumers of research. Refer to the study by Thomas et al. (2012) (Appendix A in the textbook) to answer the following questions.

1. Does the literature review identify research questions and hypotheses or answer a clinical question?

2. Is the literature review organized using a systematic approach?

3. Does the literature review use established critical appraisal criteria for specific study designs to evaluate the study for strengths, weaknesses, or limitations, as well as for conflicts or gaps in information that relate directly or indirectly to the area of interest?

4. Does the literature review provide evidence of a synthesis of the critiques that highlight the overall strengths and weaknesses of the studies reviewed and how they are similar or different between and among studies?

5. Does the literature review summarize each research or conceptual article succinctly, with appropriate references?

6. Does the literature review conclude with a summary synthesis of the reviewed material and provide recommendations for implementing the study or evidence-based practice/quality improvement project?

POSTTEST

Refer to the study by Alhusen et al. (2012) (Appendix B in the textbook) to answer the following questions.

1. What level of the 6S Pyramid is this study?

2. Next to each of the references below from Alhusen et al. (2012) in Appendix B, indicate whether it is a primary (*P*) or secondary (*S*) source AND peer-reviewed (*PR*) or not peer-reviewed (*NPR*).

    a. _____ _____   Andres, R. L., & Day, M. C. (2000). Perinatal complications associated with maternal tobacco use. *Seminars in Neonatology, 5,* 231-241.

    b. _____ _____   Cranley, M. S. (1981). Development of a tool for the measurement of maternal attachment during pregnancy. *Nursing Research, 30,* 281-284.

    c. _____ _____   Kochar, R., Fry, R., & Taylor, P. (2011). Wealth gaps rise to record highs between Whites, Blacks and Hispanics. Washington, D.C.: Pew Research Center Publications. Retrieved from: http://pewresearch. org/pubs/2069/housing-bubble-subprime-mortgageshispanics-blacks-household-wealth-disparity.

3. Does the literature review consist mainly of primary sources?

4. Does the literature review identify research questions and hypotheses or answer a clinical question?

5. Is the literature review organized using a systematic approach?

6. Does the literature review use established critical appraisal criteria for specific study designs to evaluate the study for strengths, weaknesses, or limitations, as well as for conflicts or gaps in information that relate directly or indirectly to the area of interest?

7. Does the literature review provide evidence of a synthesis of the critiques that highlight the overall strengths and weaknesses of the studies reviewed and how they are similar or different between and among studies?

8. Does the literature review summarize each research or conceptual article succinctly, with appropriate references?

9. Does the literature review conclude with a summary synthesis of the reviewed material and provide recommendations for implementing the study or evidence-based practice/quality improvement project?

REFERENCES

Alhusen, J. L., Gross, D., Hayat, M. J., et al. (2012). The influence of maternal-fetal attachment and health practices on neonatal outcome in low-income, urban women. *Research in Nursing & Health, 35,* 112-120.

DiCenso, A., Bayley, L., & Haynes, B. (2009). Accessing pre-appraised evidence: Fine tuning the 5S model into a 6S model. *Evidence-Based Nursing, 12*(4), 99-101.

Haynes, R. B. (2001). Of studies, syntheses, synopses, and systems: The "4S" evolution of services for finding current best evidence. *Evidence-Based Medicine, 6,* 36-38.

Haynes, R. B. (2007). Of studies, summaries, synopses, summaries and systems: The "5S" evolution of information services for evidence-based healthcare decisions, *Evidence-Based Nursing, 10,* 6-7.

Melvin, K. C., Gross, D., Hayat, M. J., et al. (2012). Couple functioning and post-traumatic stress symptoms in US army couples: The role of resilience. *Research in Nursing & Health, 35,* 164-177.

Thomas, M. L., Elliott, J. E., Rao, S. M., et al. (2012). A randomized clinical trial of education or motivational interviewing based coaching compared to usual care to improve cancer pain management. *Oncology Nursing Forum, 39*(1), 39-49.

4

Theoretical Frameworks for Research

INTRODUCTION

It is not uncommon for beginning consumers of research to find the theoretical part of a study to be their least favorite component. However, nursing science is the result of the interchange between research and theory. This chapter provides an overview of the use of theoretical frameworks for nursing research. An understanding of theoretical frameworks will help you examine the logical, consistent link among the theoretical framework, concepts in the study, and methods of measurement.

LEARNING OUTCOMES

On completion of this chapter, you should be able to do the following:

- Describe how a framework guides research.
- Differentiate between conceptual and operational definitions.
- Describe the relationship among theory and research and practice.
- Describe the points of critical appraisal used to evaluate the appropriateness, cohesiveness, and consistency of a framework guiding research.
- Explain the ways in which theory is used in nursing research.

Activity 1

Identify the steps the researcher must address when deciding to study a concept or construct.

1. _____

2. _____

3. _____

Activity 2

Match the definition in Column A with the appropriate term in Column B.

Column A

1. _____ A graphic or symbolic representation of a phenomenon that assists the reader to visualize the key concepts or constructs and their identified interrelationships.

2. _____ A complex concept that usually is comprised of more than one concept that is built or constructed to fit a purpose.

3. _____ Set of interrelated concepts that provides a systematic view of a phenomenon.

4. _____ Image or symbolic representation of an abstract idea.

5. _____ Defines what instruments will be used to assess the presence of the concepts and will be used to describe the amount or degree to which the concept exists.

6. _____ Goes beyond the general language meaning found in the dictionary to define or explain the meaning of a concept.

Column B

a. Theory
b. Concept
c. Conceptual definition
d. Operational definition
e. Model
f. Construct

Activity 3

The theories developed specifically by and for nurses can be classified into three categories. Identify the categories below, then identify which of the theories is the *most* abstract and which of the theories is the *least* abstract.

1. _____

2. _____

3. _____

Activity 4

In nursing research, theories are used in the research process. Identify three ways in which theories are used in the research process.

1. _____

2. _____

3. _____

Activity 5

In a study to test a theory, researchers follow certain steps. Put the following steps in sequential order from 1 (first step) to 4 (last step).

a. _____ Interprets the findings considering the predictive ability of the theory

b. _____ Chooses a theory of interest and selects a propositional statement to be examined

c. _____ Determines if there are implications for further use of the theory in practice

d. _____ Develops hypotheses that have measurable variables

Activity 6: Web-Based Activity

Access the following website:

www.jcu.edu.au/soc/nursoc/html_pages/nursing_research.htm

Go to #7, Conceptual Theoretical Frameworks, and explore the conceptual frameworks presented.

POSTTEST

Nursing theories have similarities and differences based on their scope or degree of abstraction. For questions 1 through 8, match the description in Column A with the appropriate type of nursing theory in Column B. (The type of nursing theories in Column B are used more than once, and more than one can apply to the description in Column A.)

Column A

Column B

1. _____ Composed of a limited number of concepts

2. _____ Sometimes referred to as *conceptual models*

3. _____ Focused on a limited aspect of reality

4. _____ Narrow in scope

5. _____ Most abstract level of theory

6. _____ All-inclusive conceptual structures that tend to include views on the person, health, and the environment

7. _____ Explain a small aspect of phenomena and processes

8. _____ Usually limited to specific populations or a field of practice

a. Grand
b. Situation-specific
c. Middle range

For questions 9 through 15, answer True (T) or False (F).

9. _____ Use of non-nursing theories is not important for providing evidence-based care.

10. _____ Correlational research designs are frequently used in studies that use a theory as a framework for a study.

11. _____ Beginning with theory gives a researcher a logical way of collecting data to describe, explain, and predict nursing practice.

12. _____ Certain grand theories are better than others with respect to nursing research.

13. _____ Qualitative research designs are used to test a theory.

14. _____ Theories are only used in qualitative research designs.

15. _____ Theory-generating research is inductive; it uses a process by which generalizations are developed from specific observations.

5

Introduction to Qualitative Research

INTRODUCTION

Qualitative research is a term often applied to naturalistic investigations—research that involves studying phenomena in places where they are occurring. Qualitative research approaches are based on a perceived perspective or holistic worldview that says there is not a single reality. Instead, reality is viewed as based on perceptions that differ from person to person and change over time; meaning can only be truly understood if it is associated with a specific situation or context. Qualitative research is about understanding phenomena and finding meaning through examining the pieces that make up the whole. Through different forms of qualitative nursing research methods, each method of investigation presents a unique approach to studying the phenomena of interest to nurses and the discipline.

Evidence-based practice has been primarily focused on findings that come from systematic reviews of the literature that use models examining the effectiveness of interventions. As acceptance has grown for the use of evidence-based practice in nursing, arguments about the place of qualitative research in this process have arisen. Questions of interest to nursing that have not been previously or thoroughly studied are often best investigated using qualitative methods. When new perspectives are introduced to practice, the use of qualitative investigation may be the best way to gain early understanding that can later be studied using empirical measures. However, reviews of qualitative research about a given topic can also provide meaningful insight into practice issues that can be directly applied in clinical settings.

LEARNING OUTCOMES

On completion of this chapter, you should be able to do the following:

- Describe the components of a qualitative research report.
- Describe the beliefs generally held by qualitative researchers.
- Identify four ways qualitative findings can be used in evidence-based practice.

Activity 1

Chapter 5 of the textbook provides an overview of qualitative research and introduces a variety of terms that have important implications for understanding qualitative research. Take some time to define the following terms and be sure that you can differentiate them.

a. Naturalistic settings:

b. Sample:

c. Purposive sample:

d. Recruitment:

e. Data saturation:

f. Setting:

g. Themes:

Activity 2

Compare qualitative research with quantitative research for the following steps in the research process.

	Qualitative	Quantitative
Sample recruitment		
Data collection		

Activity 3

Review Appendix C (Seiler & Moss, 2012). Find and summarize the following elements.

Element	Summary
Purpose	
Method	
Sample and setting	
Data collection	

POSTTEST

1. Identify whether each of the following beliefs reflects the quantitative or the qualitative research method.

   a. _____ Statistical explanation

   b. _____ Interviews

   c. _____ Multiple realities

   d. _____ Naturalistic setting

   e. _____ Predetermined number of participants

   f. _____ Quotations

2. Put the following components of a qualitative research report in sequential order from 1 (first step) to 7 (last step) and provide a brief description of each.

   _____ Data analysis:

   _____ Sample:

   _____ Review of the literature:

   _____ Data collection:

   _____ Study setting:

   _____ Findings:

   _____ Study design:

REFERENCE

Seiler, A., & Moss, V. A. (2012). The experiences of nurse practitioners providing health care to the homeless. *Journal of the American Academy of Nurse Practitioners, 24*, 303-312.

Qualitative Approaches to Research

INTRODUCTION

Qualitative research continues to gain recognition as a sound method for investigating the complex human phenomena less easily explored using quantitative methods. Qualitative research methods provide ways to address both the science and art of nursing. Qualitative methods are especially well-suited to address phenomena related to health and illness that are of interest to nurses and nursing practice. Nurse researchers and investigators from other disciplines are continuing to discover the value of findings obtained through qualitative studies. Nurses can be better-prepared to critique the appropriateness of a research design and identify the usefulness of the study findings when the unique differences between quantitative and qualitative research approaches are understood.

Although there are many designs for qualitative research, five methods are most commonly used by nurses. These methods are phenomenology, grounded theory, ethnography, and case study. A newer methodology known as *community-based participatory research* that is gaining increased respect from nursing scientists who are investigating behavioral phenomena is also described in this chapter. Understanding and care are concepts related to behaviors that are important to nurses in the practice of clinical nursing care in a variety of settings across the lifespan. Each of these qualitative methods allows the researcher to approach the phenomena of interest from a different perspective. Each offers the investigator a different perspective and suggests findings that address different realms of human experience.

LEARNING OUTCOMES

On completion of this chapter, you should be able to do the following:

- Identify the processes of phenomenological, grounded theory, ethnographic, and case study methods.
- Recognize appropriate use of community-based participatory research methods.
- Discuss significant issues that arise in conducting qualitative research in relation to such topics as ethics, criteria for judging scientific rigor, and combination of research methods.
- Apply critiquing criteria to evaluate a report of qualitative research.

Activity 1

Match the following definitions in Column A with the appropriate terms in Column B.

Column A

Column B

1. _____ No new data emerging

2. _____ Select experiences to help the researcher test ideas and gather complete information about developing concepts

3. _____ Outsider's view

4. _____ Identify personal biases about the phenomenon

5. _____ Insider's view

6. _____ Symbolic categories that include smaller categories

7. _____ Individuals who have special knowledge, status, or communication skills and who are willing to teach the ethnographer about the phenomenon

a. Theoretical sampling
b. Emic
c. Etic
d. Data saturation
e. Bracketed
f. Domains
g. Key informants

Activity 2

Six qualitative research methods are discussed in the textbook in relation to five basic research elements. Use your textbook to compare research elements of each of the different types of qualitative methods. Briefly describe a key aspect of each element for the different qualitative methods. This activity will assist you to compare and contrast the similarities and differences in these methods.

1. Identifying the phenomenon	
Phenomenology	
Grounded theory	
Ethnography	
Case study	
Community-based participatory research	

2. Structuring the study	
Phenomenology	
Grounded theory	
Ethnography	
Case study	
Community-based participatory research	

3. Data collection	
Phenomenology	
Grounded theory	
Ethnography	
Case study	
Community-based participatory research	

4. Data analysis	
Phenomenology	
Grounded theory	
Ethnography	
Case study	
Community-based participatory research	

5. Description of the findings	
Phenomenology	
Grounded theory	
Ethnography	
Case study	
Community-based participatory research	

Activity 3

Read the Methods section of the study by Seiler & Moss (2012) in Appendix C of the textbook and answer the following questions.

1. What research design was used to conduct this research study?

2. Describe the sample in this study.

3. What important procedures and methods were used to collect data in this study?

4. What methods were used during data analysis?

Activity 4

The five qualitative methods of research are the phenomenological, grounded theory, ethnographic, case study, and historical methods. For each characteristic listed below, indicate which method of qualitative research it describes. Use the abbreviations from the key provided. Some characteristics may be described by more than one method.

Key:

    A = Phenomenological
    B = Grounded theory
    C = Ethnographic
    D = Case study

1. _____ Uses "emic" and "etic" views of subjects' worlds
2. _____ Research questions focus on basic social processes that shape behavior
3. _____ Central meanings arise from subjects' descriptions of lived experience
4. _____ Focuses on a dimension of day-to-day existence
5. _____ Uses theoretical sampling to analyze data
6. _____ Studies the peculiarities and commonalities of a specific case
7. _____ Discovers "domains" to analyze data
8. _____ States that individuals' history is a dimension of the present
9. _____ Attempts to discover underlying social forces that shape human behavior
10. _____ Attention is given to a single case
11. _____ Interviews "key informants"
12. _____ Focuses on describing cultural groups
13. _____ Uses constant comparative method during data analysis
14. _____ Researcher "brackets" personal bias or perspective
15. _____ Can include quantitative and/or qualitative data
16. _____ Subjects are currently experiencing a circumstance
17. _____ Collects remembered information from subjects
18. _____ Involves "field work"
19. _____ May use photographs to describe current behavioral practices
20. _____ May not include exhaustive literature search
21. _____ Uses an inductive approach to understanding basic social processes

POSTTEST

For questions 1 through 5, answer True (T) or False (F).

1. _____ Qualitative research focuses on the whole of human experience in naturalistic settings.

2. _____ *External criticism in historical research* refers to the authenticity of data sources.

3. _____ In qualitative research, one would expect the number of subjects participating to be as large as those usually found in quantitative studies.

4. _____ The researcher is viewed as the major instrument for data collection.

5. _____ Qualitative studies strive to eliminate extraneous variables.

6. To what does the term *saturation* in qualitative research refer?
   a. Data repetition
   b. Subject exhaustion
   c. Researcher exhaustion
   d. Sample size

7. Data in qualitative research are often collected by which of the following procedures?
   a. Questionnaires sent out to subjects
   b. Observation of subjects in naturalistic settings
   c. Interviews
   d. All of the above

8. The qualitative method that includes an inductive approach using a systematic set of procedures to create a theory about basic social processes is known as which of the following?
   a. Phenomenology
   b. Grounded theory
   c. Ethnography
   d. Case study
   e. Community-based participatory research

9. What is the qualitative method that attempts to construct the meaning of the lived experience of human phenomena?
   a. Phenomenology
   b. Grounded theory
   c. Ethnography
   d. Case study
   e. Community-based participatory research

10. What qualitative research method would be most appropriate for studying the impact of culture on the health behaviors of urban Hispanic youth?
   a. Phenomenology
   b. Grounded theory
   c. Ethnography
   d. Case study
   e. Community-based participatory research

11. What qualitative method would be most appropriate for studying a family's experience with cystic fibrosis?
    a. Phenomenology
    b. Grounded theory
    c. Ethnography
    d. Case study
    e. Community-based participatory research

12. What qualitative method would you use to study the spread of HIV/AIDS in an urban area?
    a. Phenomenology
    b. Grounded theory
    c. Ethnography
    d. Case study
    e. Community-based participatory research

13. Which data analysis process is *not* used with grounded theory methodology?
    a. Bracketing
    b. Axial coding
    c. Theoretical sampling
    d. Open coding

REFERENCE

Seiler, A., & Moss, V. A. (2012). The experiences of nurse practitioners providing health care to the homeless. *Journal of the American Academy of Nurse Practitioners, 24,* 303-312.

Appraising Qualitative Research

INTRODUCTION

Qualitative research provides an opportunity to generate new knowledge about phenomena less easily studied with empirical or quantitative methods. Nurse researchers are increasingly using qualitative methods to explore holistic aspects less easily investigated with objective measures. In qualitative research, the data are less likely to involve numbers and most likely will include text derived from interviews, focus groups, observation, field notes, or other methods. The data tend to be mostly narrative or written words that require content rather than statistical analysis. The important contributions being made to nursing knowledge through qualitative studies make it important for nurses to possess skills that enable them to evaluate and critique qualitative research reports. This chapter describes the criteria needed to evaluate and critique qualitative research reports. Published research reports, whether they are quantitative or qualitative, must be viewed by the reviewers as having scientific merit, demonstrate rigor in the research conducted, present new knowledge, and be of interest to the journal's readers.

LEARNING OUTCOMES

On completion of this chapter, you should be able to do the following:

- Identify the influence of stylistic considerations on the presentation of a qualitative research report.
- Identify the criteria for critiquing a qualitative research report.
- Evaluate the strengths and weaknesses of a qualitative research report.
- Describe the applicability of the findings of a qualitative research report.
- Construct a critique of a qualitative research report.

Activity 1

Critiquing qualitative research enables the nurse to make sense out of the research report, build on the body of knowledge about human phenomena, and consider how the knowledge might be applicable to nursing. Learning and applying a critiquing process is the first step in this process. Column A provides examples of information from the study by Seiler and Moss (2012) found in Appendix C of the textbook. Match the information in Column A with the appropriate qualitative critical appraisal criteria in Column B. Some of the criteria in Column B are used more than once.

	Column A		**Column B**

Column A

1. _____ "Five main themes and 13 subthemes emerge from data analysis of significant statements from the nine interviews."

2. _____ "One main question was asked at the start of the interview: "Will you please describe to me your experiences in providing health care to the homeless?"

3. _____ "A qualitative naturalistic approach was utilized in this study using the principles of phenomenology to guide data collection and analysis."

4. _____ "As themes began to emerge, similar data were clustered into themes and further separated into subthemes."

5. _____ "The participants were obtained, using purposive and snowball sampling methodology, from NPs practicing for at least 6 months in southeast and northeast Wisconsin clinics that provided health care to the homeless."

6. _____ "Therefore, it was the goal of this study to address this gap in the literature in an effort to more fully understand the experiences of NPs involved in providing health care to the homeless."

7. _____ "The theme, 'how the relationship develops' and its related subthemes, 'establishing trust' and 'hearing their story' identifies ways for NPs to overcome the barriers to receiving health care perceived by homeless patients …"

8. _____ "Following each interview, audio-taped recordings were transcribed verbatim."

9. _____ "Homelessness is an increasing social and public health problem and provides unique challenges for health care professionals and the health care system."

10. _____ "Another said: 'I think the homeless community offers just tremendous opportunities to help. And for the old school nursing that I'm from, that's what a nurse is about, is to help."

11. _____ "This study helps to fill the gap in the literature and will assist health care providers to gain insight into the experience and learn what it takes to become successful in such an important and much needed role."

12. _____ "Field notes were collected."

Column B

a. Statement of phenomenon of interest
b. Purpose
c. Method
d. Sampling
e. Data collection
f. Data analysis
g. Findings
h. Discussion/ conclusions/ implications/ recommendations

Activity 2

The textbook discusses overall purposes of qualitative research. Identify the four purposes of qualitative research that the textbook identifies.

1. _____

2. _____

3. _____

4. _____

Activity 3

When critiquing a qualitative study, the following are important components of the analysis of data. Identify how you would know that the following components have been addressed in a qualitative study.

1. Credibility: _____

   _____

2. Auditability: _____

   _____

3. Fittingness: _____

   _____

Activity 4: Web-Based Activity

The Internet can be a valuable tool in gaining insight into qualitative research topics. Searching the term *qualitative research* can be a way to gain additional understanding about many aspects of this research approach. However, it is essential to identify a few quality starting points for your investigation. The University of Alberta's International Institute for Qualitative Methodology at www.ualberta.ca/~iiqm/ is an excellent place to locate information about conferences, journals, training, and international research. Start from the University of Alberta site and follow the link to the *International Journal of Qualitative Methods*. Search for the phrase *experience or theory* and note the variety of research methodologies used to explore this concept. Another good site is Judy Norris's "QualPage" at www.qualitativeresearch.uga.edu/QualPage/, a valuable resource for learning more about the various methods of qualitative research.

You may want to spend some time reviewing these websites to learn more about the state of qualitative research methods. Your instructor may want to assign some particular activities from these websites to assist you in learning about qualitative research.

POSTTEST

For questions 1 through 5, answer True (T) or False (F).

1. _____ Unlike quantitative research, prediction and control of phenomena are not the aim of qualitative research.

2. _____ Quotations are not an effective way to help the reader understand the "insider's" view.

3. _____ The goal of a published qualitative research study is to describe in as much detail as possible the "insider's" view of the phenomenon being studied.

4. _____ In a qualitative study, you should expect to find hypotheses.

5. _____ Page limitations for publishing a research study are not imposed by journals.

For questions 6 through 9, match the term in Column B with the appropriate definition in Column A.

Column A	**Column B**
6. _____ A way of describing large quantities of qualitative data in a condensed format.	a. Phenomena
	b. Meta-synthesis
7. _____ Things that are perceived by our senses.	c. Emic view
	d. Theme
8. _____ A way of integrating findings from a number of disparate qualitative investigations.	
9. _____ The view of the person experiencing the phenomenon reflective of their culture, values, beliefs, and experiences.	

REFERENCES

Norris, J. (2012, Aug 16). QualPage: Resources for qualitative research. Retrieved from www.qualitativeresearch.uga.edu/QualPage/.

Seiler, A. J., & Moss, V. A. (2012). The experiences of nurse practitioners providing health care to the homeless. *Journal of the American Academy of Nurse Practitioners, 24,* 303-312.

University of Alberta. (2001-2013). International institute for qualitative methodology. Retrieved from www.ualberta.ca/~iiqm/.

Introduction to Quantitative Research

INTRODUCTION

The phrase *research design* is used to describe the overall plan of a particular study. The design is the researcher's plan for answering specific research questions in the most accurate and efficient way possible. In quantitative research, the plan outlines how the hypotheses will be tested. The design ties together the present research problem, the knowledge of the past, and the implications for the future. Thus the choice of a design reflects the researcher's experience, expertise, knowledge, and biases.

LEARNING OUTCOMES

On completion of this chapter, you should be able to do the following:

- Define *research design*.
- Identify the purpose of research design.
- Define *control* and *fidelity* as they affect research design.
- Compare and contrast the elements that affect fidelity and control.
- Begin to evaluate what degree of control should be exercised in research design.
- Define *internal validity*.
- Identify threats to internal validity.
- Define *external validity*.
- Identify the conditions that affect external validity.
- Identify the links between the study design and evidence-based practice.
- Evaluate research design using critiquing questions.

Activity 1

Match the definitions in Column A with the research design terms in Column B. Check the glossary for help with terms.

Column A	Column B
1. _____ The antecedent variable	a. External validity
	b. Internal validity
2. _____ Sampling selection where each element has an equal chance for selection into the control or intervention group	c. Bias
	d. Research design
	e. Control
3. _____ Methods to keep the study conditions constant during the study	f. Experimental group
	g. Dependent variable
4 _____ Methods to ensure that data collection procedures remain consistent for all subjects	h. Independent variable
	i. Control group
5. _____ The vehicle for hypothesis testing or answering research questions	j. Pilot study
	k. Constancy
6. _____ Small, preliminary study	l. Randomization
7. _____ Degree to which the experimental conditions, and not uncontrolled factors, lead to the results of the study	
8. _____ Degree to which the study results can be applied to the larger population	
9. _____ Can reduce the credibility or dependability of the results of a study	
10. _____ Group that receives the treatment in a study	
11. _____ Presumed effect of the experimental variable on the outcome	
12. _____ Comparison group	

Activity 2

For each of the following situations, identify the type of threat to internal validity from the list below. Then explain the reason this is a problem, and suggest how the problem can be corrected.

History	Mortality
Instrumentation	Selection bias
Maturation	Testing

1. The researcher tested the effectiveness of a new method of teaching drug dosage and solution calculations to nursing students using a standardized calculation exam at the beginning, midpoint, and end of a 2-week course.

2. In a study of the results of a hypertension teaching program conducted at a senior center, blood pressures taken by volunteers using their personal equipment were compared before and after the program.

3. A major increase in cigarette taxes occurs during a 1-year follow-up study of the impact of a smoking cessation program.

4. The smoking cessation rates of an experimental group consisting of volunteers for a smoking cessation program were compared with the results of a control group of people who wanted to quit on their own without a special program.

5. Thirty percent of the subjects dropped out of an experimental study of the effect of a job-training program on employment for homeless women. More than 90% of the dropouts were single homeless women with at least two preschool-aged children, while the majority of subjects successfully completing the program had no preschool-aged children.

6. Nurses on a maternity unit want to study the effect of a new hospital-based teaching program on mothers' confidence in caring for their newborn infants. A survey is mailed to participants by the researchers 1 month after discharge.

Activity 3

Research design is an all-encompassing term for the overall plan to answer the research questions, including the method and specific plans to control other factors that could influence the results of the study. To become acquainted with the major elements in the design of a study, read the article by Thomas et al., 2012 (Appendix A in the textbook) and answer the following questions.

1. What was the setting for the study?_____

2. Who were the subjects? _____

3. How was the sample selected?_____

4. What were the exclusion criteria? _____

5. Were there any significant differences between the study groups? _____

_____

6. What instruments were used, and how was constancy maintained between groups?_____

_____

7. Which group served as the control group? _____

Activity 4

Now that you are familiar with a research study, use the critiquing criteria in Chapter 8 in the textbook to critique the research design of the study by Thomas et al., 2012 (Appendix A in the text). Explain your answers.

1. Is the design appropriate?

2. Is the control consistent with the research design?

3. Think about the feasibility of this study. What are some of the feasibility challenges for this study?

4. Does the design logically flow from problem, framework, literature review, and hypothesis?

5. What are the threats to internal validity, and how did the investigators control for each?

6. What are the threats to external validity, and how did the investigators control for each?

Activity 5: Web-Based Activity

Assume you are thinking about submitting a proposal for research funding to the National Institute of Nursing Research (NINR). You are a multitalented researcher and are equally qualified to conduct either qualitative or quantitative research. You are curious about the number of grants awarded that would be considered quantitative or qualitative and are interested in determining if other nurse scientists are working in your area of interest. Start at the NINR website and describe how you could use this site to get a sense of the qualitative/quantitative ratio and the topics under study.

Go to http://www.ninr.nih.gov/. Click on each of the following in order:

*   Research and Funding
*   Funded NINR Grants/Collaborative Activities
*   Follow the directions given for limiting search results to NINR-funded grants

Review the studies that appear. Do these titles give you enough information to determine if the awarded grant was qualitative or quantitative in nature? Read through the first 10 citations and label them as either qualitative or quantitative. Are any of the top 10 citations focused on your area of interest?

Note: URLs for websites may change. If you receive an error message at the URL listed above, go to your favorite search engine and type in, "National Institute for Nursing Research"; this should lead you to the desired site.

An excellent source of information about both quantitative and qualitative studies can be your own university library. Go to your campus home page and type in "library," then type in "research" or "nursing research." This can be an excellent source for full-text journals; however, they are usually password-protected, so you will need to obtain a password from your library to access them.

Activity 6: Evidence-Based Practice Activity

Review the evidence-based practice tips from Chapter 8 in the textbook. Decide which of the following statements is likely true, based on your reading, and describe how you agree or disagree with the statements.

1. If a study discusses a population of interest to you in the literature review section, but doesn't actually sample from your population of interest, that study would be useful for answering your evidence-based practice problem.

2. The study you have selected tests an intervention. The authors describe using a randomized-controlled trial design where all subjects have an equal chance to be in the control or intervention group, a manual was created to train the interventionists for this study, and there was in-person training before the intervention started that included role playing; interventions were recorded and 25% of the recordings were reviewed by the study team to assess consistency; following the intervention, subjects performed the skills taught in the intervention at the end of the teaching session and again after 3 months of performing the intervention independently. The authors do not describe specifically how they knew the subjects had received and understood the treatment (a receipt). Can you trust that these authors maintained intervention fidelity?

3. You read a study in your area of interest. The authors found that the intervention you are interested in did not produce a statistically significant result. Would you include this study?

4. You are interested in a very specific subset of a population. You are unable to find any studies that specifically sample from your population. Can you complete an evidence-based practice problem on this population?

POSTTEST

1. Review the study by Alhusen et al., 2012 (see Appendix B in the textbook). Briefly assess the major components of the research design.

   a. Use your own words to state the purpose of the study.

   b. What theoretical model did the authors base the study on?

   c. Who are the subjects?

   d. Who was excluded?

   e. What instruments were used?

   f. How do the researchers attempt to control elements affecting the results of the study?

2. Fill in the blanks by selecting from the following list of terms. Not all terms will be used.

Constancy   Mortality
Control   Internal validity
Feasibility   External validity
Selection bias   Accuracy
Reliability   History
Maturation

a. _____ is used to hold steady the conditions of the study.

b. _____ is used to describe that all aspects of a study logically follow from the problem statement.

c. The believability between this study and the world at large is known as _____.

d. The developmental, biological, or psychological processes known as _____ operate within a person over time and may influence the results of a study.

e. Time, subject availability, equipment, money, experience, and ethics are factors influencing the _____ of a study.

f. Selection bias, mortality, maturation, instrumentation, testing, and history influence the _____ of a study.

g. Voluntary (rather than random) assignment to an experimental or control condition creates a situation known as _____.

REFERENCES

Alhusen, J. L., Gross, D., Hayatt, M. J., et al. (2012). The influence of maternal-fetal attachment and health practices on neonatal outcomes in low-income women. *Research in Nursing & Health, 35,* 112-120.

National Institute of Nursing Research. Retrieved November 20, 2012 from http://ninr.nih.gov/.

Thomas, M. L., Elliott, J. E., Rao, S. M., et al. (2012). A randomized clinical trial of education or motivational interviewing based coaching compared to usual care to improve cancer pain management. *Oncology Nursing Forum, 39*(1), 39-49.

Experimental and Quasi-Experimental Designs

INTRODUCTION

This chapter contains exercises for two categories of design: experimental and quasi-experimental. These types of designs allow researchers to test the effects of nursing actions and make statements about cause-and-effect relationships. Therefore, they can be very helpful in testing solutions to nursing practice problems. However, a researcher chooses the design that allows a given situation or problem to be studied in the most accurate and effective way possible. Thus, not all problems are amenable to immediate study by these two types of design. Rather, the choice of design is dependent on the development of knowledge relevant to the problem, plus the researcher's knowledge, experience, expertise, preferences, and resources.

LEARNING OUTCOMES

On completion of this chapter, you should be able to do the following:

- Describe the purpose of experimental and quasi-experimental research.
- Describe the characteristics of experimental and quasi-experimental studies.
- Distinguish the differences between experimental and quasi-experimental designs.
- List the strengths and weaknesses of experimental and quasi-experimental designs.
- Identify the types of experimental and quasi-experimental designs.
- List the criteria necessary for inferring cause-and-effect relationships.
- Identify potential validity issues associated with experimental and quasi-experimental designs.
- Critically evaluate the findings of experimental and quasi-experimental studies.
- Identify the contribution of experimental and quasi-experimental designs to evidence-based practice.

Activity 1

Fill in the blank for each of the following descriptions with a term selected from the list of types of experimental and quasi-experimental designs. Some terms may be used more than once and not all terms may be used.

After-only	One-group
After-only nonequivalent control group	Nonequivalent control group
Experimental	Solomon four-group
True experimental	Time series

1. _____ designs are particularly suitable for testing cause-and-effect relationships because they help eliminate potential alternative explanations (threats to validity) for the findings.

2. The type of design that has two groups identical to the true experimental design, plus an experimental after-group and a control after-group is known as a(n) _____ design.

3. A research approach used when only one group is available to study for trends over a longer period of time is called a(n) _____ design.

4. The _____ design is also known as the *post-test-only control group design* in which neither the experimental group nor the control group is pretested.

5. If a researcher wants to compare results obtained from an experimental group with a control group, but was unable to conduct pretests or to randomly assign subjects to groups, the study would be known as a(n) _____ design.

6. The _____ design includes three properties: randomization, control, and manipulation.

7. When subjects are unable to be randomly assigned into experimental and control groups but are able to be pretested and posttested, the design is known as a(n) _____ design.

Activity 2

Review the study by Thomas et al. (2012) in Appendix A of the textbook, and then answer the following questions.

1. Did this study use a true experimental design? Justify your answer.

2. How does this design relate to statements about cause and effect?

3. One important condition of experimental designs is the relationship between the causal and effect variables.

   a. What are the independent variable(s)?

   b. What are the dependent variable(s)?

4. Describe some extraneous study variables that might have influenced the study findings.

Activity 3

The education department in a large hospital wants to test a program to educate and change nurse's attitudes regarding pain management. You have access to the following questionnaires: the Quick Pain Survey (QPS), the Pain Knowledge and Attitudes Questionnaire (PKQ), the Headache Assessment Tool (HAT), and the Survey on Pain in the Elderly (SPE). Your responsibility is to design a study to examine the outcome of this intervention program.

1. You decide to use a Solomon four-group design. Complete the chart below with an X to indicate which of the four groups receive the pretest and posttest pain questionnaire, and which receive the experimental teaching program.

	Pretest	Teaching	Posttest
Group A	_____	_____	_____
Group B	_____	_____	_____
Group C	_____	_____	_____
Group D	_____	_____	_____

2. How would you assign nurses to each of the four groups?

3. What would you use as a pretest for the groups receiving the pretest?

4. What is the experimental treatment?

5. What is the outcome measure for each group?

6. Based on your reading, for what types of issues is this design particularly effective?

7. What is the major advantage of this type of design?

8. What is a disadvantage of this type of design?

Activity 4

1. You may be questioning why anyone would use a quasi-experimental design if an experimental design has the advantage of being so much stronger in detecting cause-and-effect relationships and enabling the researcher to generalize the results to a wider population. In what instances might it be advantageous to use a quasi-experimental design?

2. What must the researcher do to generalize the findings from a quasi-experimental research study?

3. What must a clinician do before application of research findings into practice?

Activity 5: Web-Based Activity

In this activity, you are looking for experimental nursing research studies.

1. Use your library access to enter PubMed or go to http://www.ncbi.nlm.nih.gov/pubmed/ and type in "experimental studies nursing." How many articles were found?

2. Look at the first 10 articles. Are they actual experimental studies? If not, what are they?

3. Now navigate to the left column of the page. Find the additional filters and look at "article type" unselect any article types that are chosen and scroll to the bottom. Select only "randomized controlled trials". Next, find the "species" tab and select only "humans". How many articles were found using these limits? Do these articles differ from those found in your previous search?

4. Now go to the link for "additional filters at the bottom of the menu on the left side of the page. Select "Journal categories". Now choose only "Nursing journals". How many articles were found with this additional limit? Do they differ from your previous search?

Activity 6: Evidence-Based Practice Activity

When using evidence-based practice strategies, the first step is to decide which level of evidence a research article provides. Review Figure 1-1 in the textbook, and determine the level of evidence for each of the following.

1. A committee of neonatal experts at your local hospital issues an opinion paper

2. An advanced-practice oncology nursing society conducted an evidence-based study of systematic reviews and issued a clinical practice guideline about catheter infection prevention

3. A single phenomenological study of the lived experience of being homeless and pregnant

4. A large randomized controlled clinical trial

5. A single study that used a nonequivalent control group design

POSTTEST

1. Identify whether the following studies are (E) experimental or (Q) quasi-experimental.

   a. _____ Fifty teen mothers are randomly assigned into an experimental parenting support group and a regular support group. Before the program and at the end of the 3-month program, mother-child interaction patterns are compared between the two groups.

   b. _____ Patients on two separate units are given a patient satisfaction with care questionnaire to complete at the end of their first hospital day and on the day of discharge. The patients on one unit receive care directed by a nurse case manager, and the patients on the other unit receive care from the usual rotation of nurses. Patient satisfaction scores are compared.

   c. _____ Students are randomly assigned to two groups. One group receives an experimental independent study program and the other receives the usual classroom instruction. Both groups receive the same posttest to evaluate learning.

   d. _____ A study was conducted to compare the effectiveness of a music relaxation program with silent relaxation on lowering blood pressure ratings. Subjects were randomly assigned into groups and blood pressures were measured before, during, and immediately after the relaxation exercises.

   e. _____ Reading and language development skills were compared between a group of children with chronic otitis media and a group of children without a history of ear problems.

2. Identify the type of experimental or quasi-experimental design for each of the following examples. Use the numbers from the key provided.

Key: 1 = After-only
2 = After-only nonequivalent control group
3 = True experiment
4 = Nonequivalent control group
5 = Time series
6 = Solomon four-group

a. _____ Nurses are randomly assigned to a new self-study program or the usual ECG teaching program. Knowledge of ECGs is tested before and after the program for both groups.

b. _____ Babies who tested positive on toxicology screening at birth are randomly assigned into groups to receive either routine care or a special public health nurse intervention program. Health outcomes are tested and compared at 6 months.

c. _____ A school nurse clinic is set up at one school. Health care outcomes are measured at the end of a year from that school and compared with health outcomes at a comparable school that does not have a clinic.

d. _____ Diabetic patients were randomly assigned to either one of two control groups receiving routine home health care or to one of two groups with a new diabetic teaching program. Patients in one of the control groups and in one of the teaching groups took a test of diabetic knowledge as soon as they were assigned to a group. Patients in the other two groups were not pretested. All patients completed a posttest at the conclusion of the 3-week program.

e. _____ A new peer AIDS prevention program was implemented in one high school. A second high school without the program served as a control group. An AIDS knowledge test was administered at both schools before and after the program was completed.

f. _____ Trends in patient falls were summarized each week 1 year before and for the first year after implementation of a new hospital-based quality assurance program.

Nonexperimental Designs

INTRODUCTION

Nonexperimental designs can provide extensive amounts of data that may help fill in the gaps found in nursing research. These designs help us clarify, see the real world, and assess relationships between variables, and they can provide clues that direct future, more controlled research. In this way, experimental, quasi-experimental, and nonexperimental designs complement each other. Each provides necessary components of our knowledge base. Nonexperimental designs allow us to discover some of the territory of nursing knowledge before trying to rearrange parts of it. It can be the base on which knowledge is built and further refined with quasi-experimental and experimental research.

LEARNING OUTCOMES

On completion of this chapter, you should be able to do the following:

- Describe the overall purpose of nonexperimental designs.
- Describe the characteristics of survey, relationship, and difference designs.
- Define the differences among survey, relationship, and difference designs. List the advantages and disadvantages of surveys and each type of relationship and difference designs.
- Identify methodological and secondary analysis methods of research.
- Identify the purposes of methodological and secondary analysis methods of research.
- Describe the purposes of a systematic review, meta-analysis, integrative review, and clinical practice guidelines.
- Define the differences between a systematic review, meta-analysis, integrative review, and clinical practice guidelines.
- Discuss relational inferences versus causal inferences as they relate to nonexperimental designs.
- Identify the critical appraisal criteria used to critique nonexperimental research designs.
- Apply the critiquing criteria to the evaluation of nonexperimental research designs as they appear in research reports.
- Apply the critiquing criteria to the evaluation of systematic reviews and clinical practice guidelines.
- Evaluate the strength and quality of evidence by nonexperimental designs.
- Evaluate the strength and quality of evidence provided by systematic reviews, meta-analysis, integrative reviews, and clinical practice guidelines.

Activity 1

Determine an answer for each of the following items. Once you have an answer, study the diagram to find each answer. The words will always be in a straight line. They may be read up or down, left to right, right to left, or diagonally. When you find one of the words, draw a circle around it. Any single letter may be used in more than one word, but when the puzzle is finished, not all words will be used. There are no spaces or hyphens between the words in the puzzle, thus if it is a multiword answer, link the letters together as if it is all one word. Some of the terms will be used more than once to fill in the blanks in the statements below.

Experimental Design Puzzle

```
L  O  N  G  I  T  U  D  I  N  A  L  D  M  E
C  I  S  P  U  E  Q  W  H  X  O  I  Y  H  X
C  R  F  L  G  Y  Q  E  R  C  X  E  C  G  P
U  W  O  L  Z  S  B  Q  F  H  V  O  H  H  O
N  T  L  S  C  I  S  Z  A  R  R  O  I  U  S
L  G  T  R  S  D  L  D  U  R  Z  L  D  O  T
U  E  I  O  I  S  Q  S  E  D  L  V  W  O  F
I  U  W  S  J  J  E  L  O  S  Y  U  H  I  A
G  T  D  K  X  O  A  C  I  E  M  D  I  I  C
Q  W  R  E  E  T  O  K  T  T  E  S  T  A  T
A  S  A  M  I  K  E  N  B  I  B  H  U  L  O
D  U  O  O  K  L  H  N  P  H  O  B  Z  V  F
M  C  N  G  U  L  U  E  O  L  Y  N  R  K  C
K  A  M  F  G  U  P  Q  S  B  Z  L  A  H  T
L  W  J  F  V  N  E  W  J  S  W  L  E  L  V
```

1. This type is better known for the breadth than the depth of data collected. _____

2. A major disadvantage is the length of time needed for data collection. _____

3. The main question is whether or not variables covary. _____

4. These words mean *after the fact.* _____

5. This eliminates the confounding variable of maturation. _____

6. This quantifies the magnitude and direction of a relationship. _____

7. Collects data from the same group at several points in time. _____

8. Can be surprisingly accurate if the sample is representative. _____

9. Uses data from one point in time. _____

10. This is based on two or more naturally occurring groups with different conditions of the presumed independent variable. _____

Activity 2

Listed below are a series of advantages and disadvantages for various types of nonexperimental designs. For each type of design, pick at least one advantage (A) and one disadvantage (D) from the list that accurately describes a quality of the design. Then insert the A or D and the appropriate number in the list below.

	Advantages	Disadvantages
Correlation studies	_____	_____
Cross-sectional	_____	_____
Ex post facto	_____	_____
Longitudinal	_____	_____
Prospective	_____	_____
Retrospective	_____	_____
Survey	_____	_____

Advantages

A1 A great deal of information can be economically obtained from a large population.

A2 Ability to assess changes in the variables of interest over time.

A3 Explores relationships between variables that are inherently not manipulable.

A4 Offers a higher level of control than a correlational study.

A5 They facilitate intelligent decision-making using objective criteria to guide the process.

A6 Each subject is followed separately and serves as his own control.

A7 Stronger than retrospective studies because of the degree of control on extraneous variables.

A8 Less time-consuming, less expensive, and thus more manageable for the researcher.

Disadvantages

D1 The inability to draw a causal linkage between two variables.

D2 An alternative hypothesis could be the reason for the relationships.

D3 The researcher is unable to manipulate the variables of interest.

D4 The researcher is unable to determine a causal relationship between variables because of lack of manipulation, control, and randomization.

D5 The information obtained tends to be superficial.

D6 The researcher must know sampling techniques, questionnaire construction, interviewing, and data analysis.

D7 No randomization in sampling because preexisting groups are studied.

D8 Internal validity threats such as testing and mortality are present.

D9 Subject loss to follow-up and attrition may lead to unintended sample bias that affects external validity and generalizability of findings.

Activity 3

Each of the following are descriptions of nonexperimental studies. For each example, determine the type of design used from the list provided. Not all designs are used as examples, and some will be used more than once.

C	Correlation studies	P	Prospective
CS	Cross-sectional	R	Retrospective
E	Ex post facto	SC	Survey comparative
L	Longitudinal	SD	Survey descriptive
M	Methodological	SE	Survey exploratory
MA	Meta-analysis		

Remember, some studies use more than one type of nonexperimental design.

1. A public health education nurse working with a senior center surveyed all residents to determine their priorities for health education classes and events.

   Type of design: _____

2. A study of children ages 2-18 years with diabetes collected data every year. Information collected included health surveys, HbA1c levels, 24-hour diet recall, and measurements of height and weight. Children were assessed yearly and were included in the study up to the age of 18 years; data was collected for 10 consecutive years.

   Type of design: _____

3. A study of 200 low-income seniors, approximately half Caucasian and half African American. Explored the relationship between hypertension, depression, self-esteem, and health-seeking behaviors. The data was collected on one occasion.

   Type of design: _____

4. A study examined the relationship of maternal dietary choices and infant birth weight. Medical records of 1,000 postpartum women were examined to determine dietary choices and the relationship of a vegetarian or vegan diet with infant birth weight.

   Type of design: _____

5. An exploration of the relationship between hypertension and social interaction in elderly adults living in isolated rural areas.

   Type of design: _____

6. Forty-seven items were initially developed for the Haber and Wood Student Assessment Tool (HWSAT) after a thorough examination of the literature. These items were reviewed for relevance to the domain of content by a panel of eight experts using content validation.

   Type of design: _____

7. The purpose of this study is to examine the effect of simulation in nursing education and pass rates on board examinations. The LoBiondo-Wood Model of concept development was used in this study. An electronic search of the literature in several databases (CINAHL, MEDLINE, PubMed, Scopus) was conducted to find studies of the effectiveness of simulation on board exam pass rates in the nursing literature. The study used statistical analysis of 23 quantitative studies that met predetermined inclusion criteria to evaluate the effect of simulation on board pass rates.

Type of design: _____

Activity 4

Use the critiquing criteria from the chapter to analyze the study by Alhusen et al. (2012) (see Appendix B in the textbook). In this study, the objective was to examine relationships of maternal-fetal attachment, health practices during pregnancy, and neonatal outcomes. The sample consisted of low-income African-American women and their neonates.

1. Type of design: _____

2. Did the authors publish their hypothesis(es)? If so, what was is/are they?

3. What were the inclusion and exclusion criteria, and how do they relate to the study aims?

4. How often were data collected and when did data collection occur?

Activity 5

Review the Critical Thinking Decision Path: Nonexperimental Design Choice in the textbook. If you wanted to test a relationship between two variables in the past such as the incidence of reported back injuries of nurses working in newborn nurseries compared with those nurses working in long-term care, which design would you use?

Activity 6: Web-Based Activity

This activity will assist you in finding nursing research survey instruments if you are considering gathering data for a nonexperimental survey study. Use two search engines (Google, Google Scholar) and one website (PubMed) to find instruments, and then compare the three sources to determine which is the most helpful to you.

1. First, go to the National Library of Medicine, PubMed site at http://www.ncbi.nlm.nih.gov/pubmed/.

   You will see a box labeled "Search" with the term "PubMed" in it. The box next to it has the label "for" before it; type in "Nursing Research Survey Instruments." Click on "Go." Review the results you obtain.

   a. How many results were identified?

   b. Print the first page and review the first five citations. Do these citations give you information about the survey instruments that are available to use in nursing research?

   c. How is the information presented? Is it in a manner that is useful to planning research?

   d. How current is the information?

   e. Now place quotation marks around your search terms and search the following: nursing and research and "survey instruments". How many results were identified? Did the use of quotation marks make your search more targeted?

2. Now go to your library home page, choose a nursing database (CINAHL) or a general database (Medline, Scopus, Ebsco). Access the database and open a search page. In the box, type in "Nursing Research Survey Instruments." Click on "Search." Review the results you obtain.

   a. How many results were identified?

   b. Print the first page and review the first five citations. Do these citations differ from the first five citations on PubMed?

   c. How is the information presented? Is it in a manner that is useful to planning research?

   d. How current is the information?

Activity 7: Evidence-Based Practice Activity

1. What is the value of nonexperimental studies, such as ones that demonstrate a strong relationship in predictive correlational studies for evidence-based practice?
   a. None
   b. They provide evidence only for training purposes.
   c. They demonstrate cause-and-effect relationships and can be used in decision-making regarding changes in practice.
   d. They lend support for attempting to influence the independent variable in a future intervention study.

2. Which of the following nonexperimental designs provides a quality of evidence for evidence-based practice that is stronger than the others, because the researcher can determine the incidence of a problem and its possible causes?
   a. Cross-sectional
   b. Longitudinal cohort
   c. Survey

3. When you, the research consumer, are using the evidence-based practice model to consider a change in practice, you will initially make your decision based on the strength and quality of evidence provided by the meta-analysis. Following this, what other two characteristics will be important for you to consider? (There are two correct responses.)
   a. Clinical expertise
   b. Patient values
   c. The strength of the evidence
   d. The quality of the evidence
   e. The literature review

POSTTEST

Choose from among the following words to complete the posttest. Each word may be used one time; however, this list duplicates some words because they are used in more than one answer.

Comparative	Exploratory	Methodological	Retrospective
Correlational	Ex post facto	Prospective	Retrospective
Cross-sectional	Interrelational	Prospective	Survey
Cross-sectional	Longitudinal	Relationship-difference	Variables
Descriptive	Longitudinal	Retrospective	

1. In comparative surveys, the researcher does not manipulate the _____, but assesses data in order to provide evidence for future nursing intervention studies.

2. _____ is the broadest category of nonexperimental design.

3. The category from item #2 can be further classified as _____, _____, and _____.

4. The second major category of nonexperimental design, according to LoBiondo-Wood and Haber, includes _____ studies.

5. The researcher is using _____ design when examining the relationship between two or more variables.

6. _____ designs have many similarities to quasi-experimental designs.

7. _____ design used in epidemiological work is similar to ex post facto.

8. LoBiondo-Wood and Haber discuss three types of developmental studies. They are:

   a. _____

   b. _____

   c. _____

9. _____ studies collect data at one point in time, while _____ collects data from the same group at different points in time.

10. A(n) _____ study looks at presumed causes and moves forward in time to presumed effects.

11. The researcher is using a(n) _____ design if he or she is trying to link present events to events that have occurred in the past.

12. The _____ researcher is interested in identifying an intangible construct (concept) and making it tangible with a paper-and-pencil instrument or observation protocol.

REFERENCE

Alhusen, J. L, Gross, D., Hayat, M. J., et al. (2012). The influence of maternal-fetal attachment and health practices on neonatal outcomes in low-income, urban women. *Research in Nursing & Health, 35*(2), 112-120.

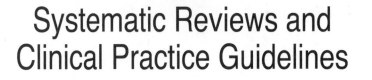

Systematic Reviews and Clinical Practice Guidelines

INTRODUCTION

Systematic reviews and clinical practice guidelines that assess multiple studies based on a single clinical question are an important element in many evidence-based practice problems. These studies provide an important means for organizing and analyzing the quality, consistency, and quantity of research findings. Thus, it is important to have an understanding of the differences between the types of systematic reviews and clinical guidelines and to develop critiquing skills, so that when you find meaningful results for your clinical question, you can have a solid foundation for understanding the conduct and content of these studies.

LEARNING OUTCOMES

On completion of this chapter, you should be able to do the following:

- Describe the types of research reviews.
- Describe the components of a systematic review.
- Differentiate among a systematic review, a meta-analysis, and an integrative review.
- Describe the purpose of clinical guidelines.
- Differentiate between an expert- and an evidence-based clinical guideline.
- Critically appraise systematic reviews and clinical practice guidelines.

Activity 1

Fill in the blanks for the following statements.

1. A(n) _____ is a form of _____; however, the statistical analysis inherent in this type of study differentiates it from other broad categories of reviews.

2. A(n) _____ is the most general category of review and synthesizes the findings of quantitative or qualitative studies without using a statistical analysis.

3. A(n) _____ provides Level I evidence.

4. Statements or recommendations that are systematically developed for clinicians are known as _____.

5. While _____ are based on the opinions of experts in a field, _____ are developed using a scientific process.

Activity 2

Think about the components of a systematic review (you may also want to refer to Box 11-1) and provide your reasoning about which components add to or fulfill the following qualities of a high-quality systematic review.

1. Clear aims:_____

   _____

2. Transparency and reproducibility: _____

   _____

3. Rigorous search: _____

   _____

4. Validity assessment:_____

   _____

5. Systematic presentation: _____

   _____

Activity 3

All of the following statements are about systematic reviews and clinical guidelines. For each statement, determine the type(s) of reviews or guidelines described by the statement and write the abbreviation for each type in the box after the statement. Each statement may be described by more than one type of review or guideline.

SR   Systematic review
MA   Meta-analysis
IR   Integrative review
ECG   Expert-based clinical guideline
EBCG   Evidence-based clinical guideline

1. A summary of studies, systematically found in the literature; focuses on a clearly stated question with a critical appraisal of the findings in a that area	
2. A method for searching and integrating the literature related to a specific clinical issue	
3. A review that uses statistical methods to assess and combine studies of the same design	
4. May review research literature, theoretical literature, or both. May include quantitative and/or qualitative research	

5. Statements or recommendations that link research and practice to guide practitioners	
6. Guidelines based on a rigorous literature search complete with an evidence table showing the quality and strength of the evidence upon which the guideline is based	
7. Can provide a precise estimate of *effect*	
8. Guidelines for areas of clinical practice without a sufficient research base, often use expert opinion and whatever research is available	
9. Could be evaluated using the AGREE II instrument to determine quality and applicability to practice	
10. The broadest category of review	
11. The Cochrane Collaboration is a large repository of these	

Activity 4: Web-Based Activity

This activity will assist you in finding a clinical guideline online.

 a. First, go to the National Center on Shaken Baby Syndrome website at www.dontshake. org.

 b. Using the tabs at the top of the page, click on "All about SBS/AHT."

 c. Using the links on the left side of the page, click on "Position statements on SBS/AHT."

 d. Following the link under "Categories" (right side of the page), click on "American Academy of Pediatrics Policy Statement."

 e. Click the link to the full policy statement.

1. What type of clinical guideline is this? What is your rationale for your answer?

2. What group was this guideline developed for?

3. What was the purpose of this guideline?

4. How does this guideline apply to clinical practice?

Activity 5: Evidence-Based Practice Activity

1. What is the value of systematic reviews in evidence-based practice? List at least three.

2. You have a strong meta-analysis and other supporting literature on your clinical question. What else do you need to consider before you might think about a change in clinical practice?

3. When you, the research consumer, are evaluating a meta-analysis to consider a change in practice, which two of the following characteristics are most important to consider when critiquing the evidence?
   a. The number of authors in the study
   b. The strength of the evidence
   c. The readability of the literature review
   d. The quality of the evidence
   e. Inclusion of patient preference in the study

4. Review Figure 1-1, Levels of evidence: Evidence hierarchy for rating levels of evidence, associated with a study's design, from your text.
   a. For each level of evidence in the left column, write in the best description in the center column from the following list: Systematic review of qualitative studies, A well-designed RCT, Single descriptive or qualitative study, Meta-analysis of RCTs, Quasiexperimental study, Opinion of authorities, Report of expert committee, Single nonexperimental study.
   b. For each level, indicate the source of evidence (A) expert opinion, (B) qualitative, (C) quantitative, (D) combination of qualitative and quantitative, or (E) anecdotal.

Level of Evidence	Description	Source
Level I		
Level II		
Level III		
Level IV		
Level V		
Level VI		
Level VII		

POSTTEST

Fill in the blanks to complete the posttest.

1. _____ is the broadest category of review.

2. A systematic review is a summary of the _____ research literature on a focused clinical question.

3. The terms _____ and _____ are often used inter-changeably, but after completing this chapter, I know that a(n) _____ uses statistical methods for the analysis of studies.

4. In a systematic review, it is important that _____ independently evaluates and critiques the studies included and _____ in the review.

5. A(n) _____ provides the _____ because it analyzes and integrates the results of many studies.

6. A meta-analysis and a systematic review include the same components, except for the _____ of the studies.

7. It is important for a consumer of the literature to evaluate systematic reviews for potential _____.

8. A(n) _____ is a graphic depiction of the results of a number of studies; it can also be called a(n) _____.

9. _____ guidelines are developed using a scientific process including a rigorous literature search, completion of an evidence table, and summary of the quality and strength of the evidence used to make each guideline. In areas without a sufficient research base, a group of experts can use their opinions and available research to develop _____.

10. A researcher who conducts a systematic review _____ conduct the studies used in the review, rather, they use data from _____ and synthesize the information following a set of systematic methods for combining evidence.

REFERENCE

National Center on Shaken Baby Syndrome. (January 15, 2013). Retrieved from www.dont-shake.org.

Sampling

INTRODUCTION

Sampling is a process of selection in which individuals, objects, animals, or events are chosen to represent the population of a study. The ideal sampling strategy is one in which the elements truly represent the population being studied while controlling for any source of bias. The specific research question(s) determine(s) the selection of the sample, variables to measure, and a sampling frame. The sampling strategies are important and should enable the choice of a sample that represents the target population and controls for bias as much as possible to ensure that the research will be valid. Reality modulates the ideal with the consideration of sampling in relation to efficiency, practicality, ethics, and availability of subjects, which can alter the ideal strategy for a given study.

LEARNING OUTCOMES

On completion of this chapter, you should be able to do the following:

- Identify the purpose of sampling.
- Define *population, sample,* and *sampling.*
- Compare a population and a sample.
- Discuss the importance of inclusion and exclusion criteria.
- Define *nonprobability* and *probability sampling.*
- Identify the types of nonprobability and probability sampling strategies.
- Compare the advantages and disadvantages of specific nonprobability and probability sampling strategies.
- Discuss the contribution of nonprobability and probability sampling strategies to strength of evidence provided by study findings.
- Discuss the factors that influence determination of sample size.
- Discuss potential threats to internal and external validity as sources of sampling bias.
- Use the critiquing criteria to evaluate the "Sample" section of a research report.

Activity 1

Write a short definition of each of the following and explain the differences between each set of words.

1. Sample: _____

   Population: _____

   Differences: _____

2. Target population: _____

   Accessible population: _____

   Differences: _____

3. Inclusion criteria: _____

   Exclusion criteria: _____

   Differences: _____

Activity 2

1. Identify the key difference between probability and nonprobability sampling.

2. Identify the category of sampling for each of the following sampling strategies. Use the abbreviations from the key provided.

   Key:
   P = Probability sampling
   N = Nonprobability sampling

   a. _____ Convenience sampling
   b. _____ Purposive sampling
   c. _____ Simple random sampling
   d. _____ Quota sampling
   e. _____ Cluster sampling
   f. _____ Stratified random sampling

Activity 6

Review the following excerpt from a study. Using the critiquing criteria listed in the text, critique the sampling process used in this study. Refer to the study by Thomas et al. (2012) in Appendix A of the textbook.

A convenience sample was obtained by recruiting patients from six outpatient oncology clinics (three Veterans Affairs [VA] facilities, one county hospital, and one community-based practice in California, and one VA clinic in New Jersey). Patients were eligible to participate if they were able to read and understand the English language, had access to a telephone, had a life expectancy longer than six months, and had an average pain intensity score of 2 or higher as measured on a 0–10 scale, with higher scores indicating more pain. Patients were excluded if they had a concurrent cognitive or psychiatric condition or substance abuse problem that would prevent adherence to the protocol, had severe pain unrelated to their cancer, or resided in a setting where the patient could not self-administer pain medication (e.g., nursing home, board and care facility). The study was approved by the institutional review board and research committee at each of the sites. To test the interaction of time (change in scores from pre- to post-study) by assignment to the three treatment groups (i.e., control, education, or coaching), a sample size of 240 was needed to detect a medium effect (f = 0.25; h2 = 6% of explained variance). As shown in Figure 1, of the 1,911 patients who were screened, 406 were eligible to participate, 322 provided written informed consent, and 289 completed baseline assessments after being randomized to one of three groups.

1. Have the sample characteristics been completely described? Explain your answer.

2. Briefly state a description of the target population.

3. What were the major cancer diagnoses represented in the sample?

4. Were men and women equally represented?

5. Are criteria for eligibility in the sample specifically identified?

6. Have sample delimitations been established? Explain your answer.

7. How was the sample selected?

8. What kind of bias, if any, is introduced by this method?

9. Is the sample size appropriate? How is it substantiated?

10. Are there indications that the rights of the subjects have been ensured?

Activity 7: Web-Based Activity

Go to the U.S. Census website at http://www.census.gov. Click on "Quick Facts" at the left-hand side of the screen. In the box where it states, "To begin, select a state from this list or use the map," choose your home state from the drop-down menu. Click on the "Go" button.

1. Under your state's Quick Facts, look at the item titled, "White persons, percent" and write down that percent.

2. Now look for the item titled, "Black persons, percent." Write down that percent.

3. How are these groups defined? (Hint: click on the *i* on the left side of the screen.)

4. Now go back to Activity 4. Review the sample percents in the Melvin et al. (2012) study for white and black people. Are they the same as they are in the census data? Would the sample percents for black and white in the Melvin et al. study be representative of the population in your state?

Activity 8: Evidence-Based Practice Activity

The text defines *evidence-based practice* as the integration of best research evidence with clinical expertise and patient values. Evidence-based practice allows nurses to use research findings to make decisions to improve practice. Teams of nurses are applying multiple study findings to improve practice outcomes with individuals, families, and other health care professionals. Through this practice, more effective patient teaching and quality care are being realized.

13

Legal and Ethical Issues

INTRODUCTION

Patient advocacy is one of the primary roles of a professional nurse. Nowhere is this more important than in the field of research. The nurse must be a patient advocate, whether acting as the researcher, a participant in data-gathering, a provider of care for research subjects, or a research consumer. A multitude of legal and ethical issues exist in research; nurses must be aware of, assess, act on, and evaluate these issues. In addition, nurses need to be knowledgeable about the purpose and functions of the institutional review board (IRB) and the federal regulations on which they are based.

LEARNING OUTCOMES

On completion of this chapter, you should be able to do the following:

- Describe the historical background that led to the development of ethical guidelines for the use of human subjects in research.
- Identify the essential elements of an informed consent form.
- Evaluate the adequacy of an informed consent form.
- Describe the institutional review board's role in the research review process.
- Identify populations of subjects who require special legal and ethical research considerations.
- Appreciate the nurse researcher's obligations to conduct and report research in an ethical manner.
- Describe the nurse's role as patient advocate in research situations.
- Critique the ethical aspects of a research study.

Activity 1

Fill in the blanks with the correct term from the following list (not all of the terms will be used).

Beneficence   Justice
Confidentiality   Nursing research committee
Expedited review   Unauthorized research
Institutional review board   Unethical research study
HIPAA

1. _____ reviews proposals for scientific merit and congruence with the institutional policies and missions.

2. _____ reviews research proposals to assure protection of the rights of human subjects.

3. The idea that human subjects should be treated fairly and should not be denied a benefit to which the subject is entitled is _____.

4. A study of existing data that is of minimal risk to subjects may be a candidate for a(n) _____.

5. The U.S. Public Health Service studied the effects of untreated syphilis on African-American sharecroppers in Tuskegee, Alabama, and withheld penicillin treatment even after penicillin was commonly available. This is considered a(n) _____.

6. Regulation requires the health care profession to protect privacy of patient information and create standards for electronic data exchange _____.

Activity 2

List the three ethical principles relevant to the conduct of research involving human subjects. These were included in the Belmont Report (1979) and formed the basis for regulations affecting research sponsored by the federal government.

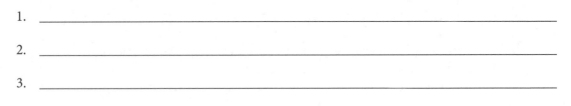

1. _____

2. _____

3. _____

Activity 3

Read the following example of a research consent form. Then review the list of the elements of informed consent that follows the example. For each item in the list of elements of informed consent, put either a "√" if the element is included in the consent or a "0" if it is absent from the consent. Summarize your findings in a paragraph at the end of the exercise.

Research Consent Form

Agreement to Participate in Research

Responsible Investigator: Mary Jo Gorney-Moreno, PhD, Professor, Nursing

Title of Protocol: A web-based interactive program to engage nurses in learning principles of pain management

We are recruiting nursing students to test a web-based interactive program to engage nurses in learning principles of pain management. There are three learning outcomes for this program, to teach: (1) appropriate and safe control of the patient's pain, (2) prevention and management of side effects of pain management, and (3) to provide accurate and complete patient teaching regarding pain and side effect management. At the end of the simulation, you will receive 3 scores, one for how well you managed patient care in each of these areas. It will take about 30 minutes to complete the simulation. The simulation is available online at http://www.cdl.edu/painless. You can complete the simulation as many times as you like; each time you will be presented with a new set of variables for the patient, Mr. Sanchez. The variables are programmed to appear randomly. We hope that this activity will enhance your knowledge related to providing pain management for your patients. There are no known risks for participation.

If you agree to participate, we welcome you and would like you to complete a pre- and post-test, as well as a short evaluation form after you complete the simulation. Your participation is voluntary, and you may withdraw at any time and for any reason. There is no penalty for not participating or withdrawing. The personal benefits for participation include assisting faculty and yourself to understand more about the effectiveness of this innovative educational intervention and to increase your knowledge. There are no costs to you or any other party.

I will ask you to print a copy of your scores from the simulation, and complete the pre- and posttest and a short questionnaire. All data collected will be coded using a unique five-character string and will not be identified with you personally. There is no risk to you.

Dr. Mary Jo Gorney-Moreno, Professor, School of Nursing, San Jose State University, is conducting this study. Dr. Gorney-Moreno can be reached at 408-555-1000. You should understand that your participation is voluntary and that choosing not to participate in this study, or in any part of this study, will not affect your relations with San Jose State University. You may refuse to participate in the entire study or in any part of the study; you are free to withdraw at any time without any negative effect on your relations with San Jose State University. The results of this study may be published, but any information that could result in your identification will remain confidential. If you have questions about this study, I will be happy to talk with you. I can be reached at 408-555-1000. If you have questions or complaints about research subjects' rights, or in the event of a research-related injury, please contact Serena Smith, PhD, Associate Vice President for Graduate Studies and Research, at (408) 555-1000.

This project has been reviewed and approved according to the San Jose State University Human Subjects Institutional Review Board procedures governing human subjects research.

Your signature indicates that you have been fully informed of your rights and voluntarily agree to participate in this study. You will be given a copy of this signed form.

By signing this form, I agree to participate in this study.

_____   _____

Subject's Signature   Date

Elements of Informed Consent

1. _____   Title of protocol
2. _____   Invitation to participate
3. _____   Basis for subject selection
4. _____   Overall purpose of the study
5. _____   Explanation of benefits
6. _____   Description of risks and discomforts
7. _____   Potential benefits
8. _____   Alternatives to participation
9. _____   Financial obligations
10. _____   Assurance of confidentiality
11. _____   In case of injury compensation
12. _____   HIPAA disclosure
13. _____   Subject withdrawal
14. _____   Offer to answer questions
15. _____   Concluding consent statement
16. _____   Identification of investigators

Activity 4

Nurses must be aware of populations that require special legal and ethical considerations. List at least four groups of subjects who are vulnerable or have diminished autonomy and thus require extra protection as research subjects.

1. _____

2. _____

3. _____

4. _____

Activity 5

Match the violation of ethical principle described from the following list with the examples presented below. More than one violation may have occurred in the examples that are cited. List all that were violated.

    a.   Degree of risk outweighed benefits
    b.   Subjects not informed they could withdraw from study at any time
    c.   Subjects not informed or offered the effective treatment that was available
    d.   Lack of informed consent
    e.   No evidence of IRB approval prior to start of research
    f.   Right to fair treatment and protection
    g.   Principles of informed consent violated or incomplete disclosure of potential risk, harm, results or side effects was given

1.   Write the letter(s) describing violation after the description of the study.

UCLA Schizophrenic Medication Study—A 1983 study examining the effects of withdrawing psychotropic medications of 50 patients under treatment for schizophrenia. Twenty-three subjects suffered severe relapses after their medications were stopped. The goal of the study was to determine if some schizophrenics might do better without medications that had deleterious side effects. Patients were not informed that their symptoms could worsen or about the severity of a potential relapse. _____

2.   List the letter(s) that correspond(s) to the ethical violation(s) listed.

The United States Public Health Service conducted a study from 1932-1973 on two groups of poor African-American male sharecroppers. One group had untreated syphilis and the other did not. Treatment was withheld from the group diagnosed with syphilis, even after it became generally available and known to be effective. Steps were taken to prevent infected subjects from obtaining penicillin. The researchers wanted to study the effects of untreated syphilis. _____

Activity 6

This activity assesses the utilization of procedures for protecting basic human rights. Review the articles in Appendices A through D of the text. For each article, describe how informed consent was obtained, and whether the author described obtaining permission from the institutional review board.

1.   Thomas et al. (2012): _____

_____

_____

2.   Alhusen et al. (2012): _____

_____

_____

3. Seiler & Moss (2012): _____

_____

_____

4. Melvin et al. (2012):_____

_____

_____

Activity 7: Web-Based Activity

Visit www.dontshake.org.

1. Identify the source of this website.

2. What populations are served by this organization?

3. What are some special legal and ethical research considerations for this population?

Activity 8: Evidence-Based Practice Activity

You are a nurse working in a postpartum unit. If you decided to make a change in your practice based on an evidence-based practice article, but first wanted to check to be certain that no misconduct had occurred in the conduct or reporting of the study, where would you find this information?

POSTTEST

1. It is necessary for researchers and nurses to protect the basic human rights of vulnerable groups. Can research studies be conducted with these populations?

   Yes, because _____

   No, because _____

2. A researcher must receive IRB approval (before / after) beginning to conduct research involving humans.

3. If you question whether a researcher has permission to conduct a study in your hospital, which documents would you want to see that demonstrate approval from which group(s)?

   _____

4. Should a researcher list all the possible risks and benefits of a participating in a research study even if some people may refuse because these items are listed in detail?

   Yes   No

5. If you agreed to collect data for a researcher who had not asked the patient's permission to participate in the research study, you would be violating the patient's right to

   _____.

6. What are two of the risks of scientific fraud or misconduct? _____

   _____

14

Data Collection Methods

INTRODUCTION

Observe, probe
Details unfold
Let nature's secrets
Be stammeringly retold.

—Goethe

The focus of this chapter is basic information about data collection. As a consumer of research, the reader needs the skills to evaluate and critique data collection methods in published research studies. To achieve these skills, it is helpful to have an appreciation of the process or the critical thinking "journey" the researcher has taken to be ready to collect the data. Each of the preceding chapters represented important preliminary steps in the research planning and designing phases prior to data collection. Although most researchers are eager to begin data collection, the planning for data collection is very important. The planning includes identifying and prioritizing data needs, developing or selecting appropriate data collection tools, and selecting and training data collection personnel before proceeding with actual collection of data.

The five types of data collection methods differ in their basic approach and in the strengths and weaknesses of their characteristics. Readers should be prepared to ask questions about the appropriateness of the measures chosen by the researcher to gather data about the variable of concern. This includes determining the objectivity, consistency, quantifiability, observer intervention, and/or obtrusiveness of the chosen data collection method.

LEARNING OUTCOMES

On completion of this chapter, you should be able to do the following:

- Define the types of data collection methods used in nursing research.
- List the advantages and disadvantages of each data collection method.
- Compare how specific data collection methods contribute to the strength of evidence in a research study.
- Identify potential sources of bias related to data collection.
- Discuss the importance of intervention fidelity in data collection.
- Critically evaluate the data collection methods used in published research studies.

Activity 1

Review each of the articles referenced below. Be especially thorough in reading the sections that relate to data collection methods. Answer the questions in relation to what you understand from the article. For some questions, there may be more than one answer.

Study 1

Thomas et al., 2012 (in Appendix A of the textbook).

1. Which data collection method(s) is/are used in this research study?
   a. A physiological measure
   b. An observational measure
   c. An interview measure
   d. A questionnaire measure
   e. Records of available data

2. In your opinion, what would be the advantage in using this(these) method(s)? What explanation do the investigators provide?

Study 2

Alhusen et al., 2012 (in Appendix B of the textbook).

1. Which data collection method is used in this research study?
   a. A physiological measure
   b. An observational measure
   c. An interview measure
   d. A questionnaire
   e. Records of available data

2. Rationale for appropriateness of data collection method:

Study 3

Seiler & Moss, 2012 (in Appendix C of the textbook).

1. What data collection method is used in this research study?
   a. A physiological measure
   b. An observational measure
   c. An interview measure
   d. A questionnaire
   e. Records of available data

2. What were the strengths of using this method?

Study 4

Melvin et al., 2011 (in Appendix D of the textbook).

1. What data collection method is used in this research study?
   a. A physiological measure
   b. An observational measure
   c. An interview measure
   d. A questionnaire
   e. Records of available data

2. Describe the data collection.

3. What are two possible problems with self-report methods that might have affected the responses given by participants? How did the researchers try to be sensitive to trauma and obtain accurate responses?

Activity 2

Using the content of Chapter 14 in the textbook, have fun completing a word-search exercise. Answer the questions below, and find the words in the puzzle.

1. Baccalaureate-prepared nurses are _____ of research.

2. _____ methods use technical instruments to collect data about patients' physical, chemical, microbiological, or anatomical status.

3. _____ is the distortion of data as a result of the observer's presence.

4. _____ are best used when a large response rate and an unbiased sample are important.

5. _____ data collection method is subject to problems of availability, authenticity, and accuracy.

6. _____ measurements are especially useful when there are a finite number of questions to be asked and the questions are clear and specific.

7. Essential in the critique of data collection methods is the emphasis on the appropriateness, _____, and _____ of the method employed.

8. _____ raises ethical questions (especially informed consent issues); therefore, it is not often used in nursing.

9. _____ _____ is the consistency of observations between two or more observers.

10. _____ is the process of translating the concepts/variables into measurable phenomena.

11. _____ is a format that uses closed-ended items, and there are a fixed number of alternative responses.

12. _____ is the method for objective, systematic, and quantitative description of communications and documentary evidence.

13. This exercise is supposed to be _____!

```
D E L I V E R S T A T I S T C S Y E S P A S
S S A C A B I N E T F O R K A Z O S P E I O
I A W O P E R A T I O N A L I Z A T I O N B
G T S N O R N E V E R B Y D N E A U X B T J
N S Y S T E M A T I C A J H T B S D V S E E
I F L I K E R T S C A L E E R R O Y A E R C
F A K S C A L E S N O V N O C A A U L R R T
H C U T A C R A T I M A P V E T P U I V A I
Y T B E B H I R T E M A H V W K I C D A T V
P C O N T E N T A N A L Y S I S P V O T E I
R O Y C B K D S I S R T S A D V A N E I R T
E R E Y O D U G K A T P I B I O I O G O R Y
A V S I B R Q U E S T I O N N A I R E N E C
C I A R E S E A R C H L L R E A C E S O L O
T O B M E X C E L A E O O D A T A C O V I N
I U E A E V A L I D S T G N O S T O O E A S
V N Y E S S I N T E R V I E W S A R F R B U
I H A P P I E N E S S P C A T A G D U N I M
T X C I T E D E L P H I A T O T P S N V L E
Y C E A T U B B S A N D L D O N N M A R I R
Y A B L E A C O N C E A L M E N T O O T T R
A I K E V A L I K E I I A B C O N S U M Y S
```

Activity 3

You are reviewing a study, and concealment is necessary; in other words, there is no other way to collect the data, and the data collected will not have negative consequences for the subject.

1. Name at least one population where concealment is not uncommon.

2. How would you obtain subjects' consent?

3. What is the major reason for using concealment?

Activity 4

You are asked to participate in discussions about impending research in your community. The purpose of the study is to identify the health status, beliefs, practices, preventive services currently known and used, and accessibility/availability of health service needs for the residents of your rural community.

In your critical thinking journey, describe what you would consider in the selection of a data collection method. Review each method and discuss the pros and cons for choosing a specific data collection method. State your rationale for your final selection. What would be your thinking about instruments and types?

Activity 5

Using the content of Chapter 14 in the textbook, circle the correct response for each question. Some questions will have more than one answer.

1. What is a primary advantage of physiological measures?
   a. The measuring tool never affects the phenomena being measured.
   b. It is one of the easiest types of methods to implement.
   c. It is unlikely that study participants/subjects can distort the physiological information.
   d. Their objectivity, sensitivity, and precision
   e. All of the above

2. Self-report measures are usually more useful than observation measures in obtaining information about which of the following?
   a. Socially unacceptable or private behaviors
   b. Complex research situations when it is difficult to separate processes and interactions
   c. When the researcher is interested in character traits
   d. All of the above

3. Which of the following would be considered disadvantages of using observational data collection methods?
   a. Individual bias may interfere with the data collection.
   b. Ethical concerns may be increasingly significant to researchers using observational data collection methods.
   c. Individual judgments and values influence the perceptions of the observers.
   d. All of the above

4. In nursing research, when might questionnaires be used as an appropriate method for data collection?
   a. Whenever expense is a concern for the researcher
   b. When a researcher is interested in obtaining information directly from the subjects
   c. When the researcher needs to collect data from a large group of subjects who are not easily accessible
   d. When accuracy is of the utmost importance to the researcher

5. Which of the following would be considered advantages of using existing records or available data to answer a research question?
   a. The use of available data reduces the risk of researcher bias in data collection.
   b. Time involvement in the research study can be reduced by the use of available records or data.
   c. Consistent collection of information over periods of time allows the researcher to study trends.
   d. All of the above

Activity 6: Web-Based Activity

Go to your library home page. Select your favorite database (some to try: PubMed, Scopus, CINAHL, Medline). Open the database and search for the following terms: "nursing assessment" AND "tool" AND "development."

How many nursing-specific assessment tools can you identify in the first 20 citations? What was the focus of the different tools? Did you see any tools you are familiar with?

Now choose an area of nursing that you are interested in and search for data measurement tools in that area. Some potential topics include fall prevention, pressure ulcers, depression, infection, anxiety, quality of life, pain, and satisfaction.

Activity 7: Evidence-Based Practice Activity

Check the evidence-based practice resources available at your clinical site or go to your library home page. Find the Cochrane Library or any database with access to evidence-based resources. Search for "nursing intervention." Choose a recent study of a nursing intervention you might use in your practice.

1. What were some of the methods used in studies included in this review? Were the methods appropriate?

2. Would you change your practice based on the evidence provided in this study? Explain your answer.

3. After looking at the Results and Discussion sections of the article you reviewed, how would you improve the data collection methods of the studies under review to strengthen the evidence?

POSTTEST

Read each question thoroughly and then circle the correct answer.

1. What is the process of translating concepts that are of interest to the researcher into observable and measurable phenomena?
   a. Objectivism
   b. Systematization
   c. Subjectivism
   d. Operationalization

2. Answering research questions pertaining to psychosocial variables can best be answered by using which data-gathering technique(s)?
   a. Observation
   b. Interviews
   c. Questionnaires
   d. All of the above

3. Collection of data from each subject in the same or in a similar manner is known as
   a. repetition.
   b. dualism.
   c. consistency.
   d. recidivism.

4. Consistency of observations between two or more observers is known as
   a. intrarater reliability.
   b. interrater reliability.
   c. consistency reliability.
   d. repetitive reliability.

5. Physiological and biological measurement might be used by nurse researchers when studying which of these variables? (Select all that apply.)
   a. A comparison of student nurses' ACT scores and their GPAs
   b. Hypertensive clients' responses to a stress test
   c. Children's dietary patterns
   d. The degree of pain relief achieved following guided imagery

6. Scientific observations should fulfill which of the following conditions?
   a. Observations are consistent with the study objectives.
   b. Observations are standardized and systematically recorded.
   c. Observations are checked and controlled.
   d. All of the above

7. In a research study, a participant observer spent regularly scheduled hours in a homeless shelter and occasionally stayed overnight. The people staying in the home were told that this person was conducting a research study. The researcher freely engaged in conversation and openly observed the homeless. What is the observational role of the researcher?
   a. Concealment without intervention
   b. Concealment with intervention
   c. No concealment without intervention
   d. No concealment with intervention

8. In unstructured observation, which of the following might occur? (Select all that apply.)
   a. Extensive field notes are recorded.
   b. Subjects are informed what behaviors are being observed.
   c. The researcher frequently records interesting anecdotes.
   d. All of the above

9. Which of the following is *not* consistent with a Likert scale?
   a. It contains closed-ended items.
   b. It contains open-ended items.
   c. It contains lists of statements.
   d. Items are evaluated on the amount of agreement.

10. Although it is acceptable to use multiple instruments within a research study, the study is more acceptable if only one method is used for the data collection.
    a. True
    b. False

11. Social desirability is seldom a concern for researchers when the data collection method used in the study is interviews.
    a. True
    b. False

12. A researcher desires to use a questionnaire in a study but cannot find one that will gather the information desired about a particular variable. The decision is made to develop a new instrument. Which of the following should the researcher do?
    a. Define the construct, formulate the items, and assess the items for content validity
    b. Develop instructions for users and pilot the instrument
    c. Estimate reliability and validity
    d. All of the above

13. The researcher who invests significant amounts of time in the development of an instrument has a professional responsibility to publish the results.
    a. True
    b. False

14. To evaluate the adequacy of various data collection methods, which of the following should be observed in the written research report?
    a. Clear identification of the rationale for selecting a physiological measure
    b. The problems of bias and reactivity are addressed with observational measures
    c. There is a clear explanation of how interviews were conducted and how interviewers were trained
    d. All of the above

15. In conducting a research study, the researcher has a responsibility to ensure that all study subjects received the same information and data was collected from all participants in the same manner.
    a. True
    b. False

REFERENCES

Alhusen, J. L., Gross, D., Hayat, M. J., et al. (2012). The influence of maternal-fetal attachment and health practices on neonatal outcome in low-income, urban women. *Research in Nursing & Health, 35,* 112-120.

Melvin, K. C., Gross, D., Hayat, M. J., et al. (2012). Couple functioning and post-traumatic stress symptoms in US Army couples: The role of resilience. *Research in Nursing & Health, 35,* 164-177.

Seiler, A., & Moss, V. A. (2012). The experiences of nurse practitioners providing health care to the homeless. *Journal of the American Academy of Nurse Practitioners, 24,* 303-312.

Thomas, M. L., Elliott, J. E., Rao, S. M., et al. (2012). A randomized clinical trial of education or motivational interviewing based coaching compared to usual care to improve cancer pain management. *Oncology Nursing Forum, 39*(1), 39-49.

15

Reliability and Validity

INTRODUCTION

If a friend tells you, "Hey, I found a new restaurant that you will really love," you will consider that information from at least two perspectives before you spend your money there. First, does this person understand your taste in food? Second, has this person given you good information about food in the past?

You answer "no" to the first question. You prefer seafood served in an elegant setting, and your friend prefers pizza served in a place with sawdust on the floor. Using this information, you will consider your friend's opinion to be invalid for you. You will never give this restaurant another thought.

But if you answer "yes" to the first question because you share similar tastes in food, you will move on to the second question. You remember the tough fettuccini, the superb Southern fried chicken, the unbaked pizza dough, and the hockey-puck biscuits from earlier recommendations. It is likely that while you and your friend share food preferences, her information is not reliable. You can't trust her to give you good information over time. If you are feeling like an adventure, you may try the new restaurant or you may not.

Validity and reliability of the data collection instruments used in a study are to be regarded in the same way that you would consider your friend's advice about restaurants. Is the instrument valid? Does it provide me with accurate information? Is the instrument reliable? Does it provide me with consistent information whenever it is used? Consideration of both validity and reliability influences your confidence in the results of the study.

LEARNING OUTCOMES

On completion of this chapter, you should be able to do the following:

- Discuss how measurement error can affect the outcomes of a research study.
- Discuss the purposes of reliability and validity.
- Define *reliability*.
- Discuss the concepts of stability, equivalence, and homogeneity as they relate to reliability.
- Compare and contrast the estimates of reliability.
- Define *validity*.
- Compare and contrast content, criterion-related, and construct validity.
- Identify the criteria for critiquing the reliability and validity of measurement tools.

- Use the critiquing criteria to evaluate the reliability and validity of measurement tools.
- Discuss how evidence related to reliability and validity contributes to the strength and quality of evidence provided by the findings of a research study and applicability to practice.

Activity 1

Either random error (*R*) or systematic error (*S*) may occur in a research study. For each of the following examples, identify the type of measurement error and how the error might be corrected.

1. _____ The scale used to obtain daily weights was inaccurate by 3 lbs. less than actual weight.

   Correction: _____

2. _____ Students chose the socially acceptable responses on an instrument to assess attitudes toward AIDS patients.

   Correction: _____

3. _____ Confusion existed among the evaluators on how to score the wound healing.

   Correction: _____

4. _____ The subjects were nervous about taking the psychological tests.

   Correction: _____

Activity 2

Validity is the extent to which a measurement tool actually measures the concepts it is supposed to measure. Use the terms from the following list to complete each of the items in this activity. (Not all terms will be used, and some terms may be used more than once.)

Concurrent validity	Content validity	Contrasted groups
Construct validity	Convergent validity	Criterion-related validity
Divergent validity	Content validity index	Factor analysis
Hypothesis testing	Multitrait-multimethod approach	Predictive validity
Context experts	Face validity	

1. _____ of the instrument was evaluated by exploratory factor analysis (EFA) and confirmatory factor analysis (CFA). Samples sizes for EFA and CFA were 632 and 578, respectively.

2. _____ is a rudimentary type of validity testing where colleagues, experts, or subjects read the instrument to evaluate if it reflects the concept the researcher is trying to measure.

3. "_____ was established by clinical experts and pregnant women" (Alhusen et al., 2012).

4. The authors and six doctoral students developed a one-page questionnaire entitled "Travel Health." Occupational health nurses ($n = 10$) with graduate-level training and experience in travel health rated the scale's items for relevance to the construct and a _____ was calculated using the average of the responses from the experts.

5. The current study showed that when the Fatigue Symptom Scale and the TIRED Scale were given to the same subjects and a correlational analysis was performed, there was _____ based on the positive correlation between both measures of the concept of fatigue.

6. Construct validity, an assessment of the relationship between the instrument and the underlying theory, can be measured in several ways. List three of these: _____, _____, and _____.

7. An instrument is being developed to measure physical activity in knee injury patients. The instrument was administered to a group of patients the day before surgery and another group of patients 6 months after surgery. A t-test found significant differences between the groups. This is a _____ test of construct validity.

Activity 3

An instrument is considered reliable if it is accurate and consistent. If the concept being studied is stable, the same results should occur when measurement is repeated.

1. Three concepts related to reliability include _____, _____, and _____.

2. Give an example of each of the two types of tests for stability.

3. In what instance would it be better to use an alternate form rather than a test-retest measure for stability?

4. Homogeneity is a measure of internal consistency. All items on the instrument should be complementary and measure the same characteristic or concepts. For each of the following examples, identify which of the following tests for homogeneity is described:

(1) Item-total correlations
(2) Split-half reliability
(3) Kuder-Richardson (KR-20) coefficient
(4) Cronbach's alpha

a. _____ The odd items of the test had a high correlation with the even numbers of the test.

b. _____ Each item on the test using a 5-point Likert scale had a moderate correlation with every other item on the test.

c. _____ Each item on the test ranged in correlation from 0.62 to 0.89 with the total.

d. _____ Each item on the true-false test had a moderate correlation with every other item on the test.

5. Review the following information about one of the instruments used in the study in Appendix D of the text: "Post-traumatic stress symptoms (PTSS). For this study, PTSS was operationalized as an individual's endorsement of symptom items on the PTSD Checklist (PCL), including problems with sleep, avoidance, memory, concentration, emotional connections, or mood. This measure consists of 17 items, scored on a 5-point Likert-type scale, regarding severity of various symptoms diagnostic of PTSD. The PCL has been widely used in both military and civilian populations to measure the prevalence of presumed PTSD and for group comparisons on levels of PTSS. Cronbach's α reliabilities have ranged from 0.92 in civilians to 0.97 in military populations. Validity has been supported by the statistically significant correlations between PCL scores and the Clinician-Administered PTSD Scale. The PCL scores range from 17 to 85, with higher scores indicative of greater PTSS. Recent research supports a clinical cut-off of 30 when used in military primary care settings to screen for levels of PTSS high enough to cause interpersonal problems. In many studies, the clinical cut-off of 50 has been used. Although the higher cut-off is more specific to the diagnosis of PTSD, we chose to use the more sensitive lower number for this study, to capture more variability in levels of PTSS. The Cronbach's α was 0.96 in our sample."

a. What is a Likert scale? How would you expect items on the PCL to look based on your knowledge of a Likert-type scale?

b. What information is given to the reader about the PCL?

c. How does this information influence your level of confidence in the results of this study?

Activity 4: Web-Based Activity

In this activity you will complete a search for instruments used to measure a nursing concept of interest to you. For this search you will use the PubMed database. You can complete the search even without library access; you just may have difficulty accessing the contents of the articles you find. Start at your library webpage and access PubMed or go to www.ncbi.nlm.nih.gov/pubmed. If you have never completed a search using MeSH terms, follow the link to the MeSH database from the PubMed main page to learn more about MeSH terms and follow the link to "help" with using MeSH. Most good searches use more than one MeSH term.

1. Think of a nursing concept you are interested in, and look it up in the MeSH database to determine if there is a different term or multiple terms used to describe this concept.

2. Search for your term combined with one or two of the following terms to find instruments related to your interest (choose the terms closest to your interest): psychometrics, questionnaires, outcome assessment, pain measurement, checklist, assessment, health care survey, health survey, validation studies, process assessment, patient satisfaction, methodology (or any other term you can think of). If you find too many results, try adding another search

term to narrow your search. If you find no results or a few results that don't match your interest, try to make your search less specific (use the MeSH dictionary to find a term less specific than your term using the MeSH categories and subheadings).

3. If you know of an instrument you are interested in, search for it by name.

4. Find the psychometric studies related to your instrument by searching for the following terms or search strings combined with the name of the instrument you have found: (reliability or reproducib* or inter rate or interrater or valid* or test retest or predictive or psychometric*) measure* (i.e., measures, measurement), assess* (i.e., assessment, assessed), self-report, exercise, valid* (i.e., valid, validation, validity), reliab* (i.e., reliable, reliability), reproducible. Your search should include titles, abstracts, keywords, and full texts.

5. Review what you have found on the reliability and validity of your instrument with what you have learned in this chapter. Is this a well-validated instrument or a new instrument with little testing?

6. If you had trouble completing your search, find a class offered by your medical library or work with a librarian to learn how to use PubMed.

Activity 5

In this activity, you will use the critiquing criteria listed in Chapter 15 of the text to think about the Thomas et al. study in Appendix A of the text.

1. How many instruments for data collection were used in this study?

2. For the Functional Assessment of Cancer Therapy–General (FACT-G):

   a. What information on validity was included in the article?

   b. Did the authors report on any tests of reliability?

   c. Name some appropriate tests of reliability for this instrument.

   d. Would a Kuder-Richardson-20 test be a good test of reliability? Why or why not?

   e. Has this instrument been previously used in this population?

    f.   If you wanted information on validity, where would you look?

    g.   Where in the article would you look to see how the results of this study compared with FACT-G scores from other studies?

Activity 6: Evidence-Based Practice Activity

Now think about the Alhusen et al. (2012) study. Look at the reliability and validity measures of the instruments used in the study. Assume you are a nurse who cares for neonates and their mothers. How would you use the results of this study to guide your practice?

POSTTEST

Using the following terms, complete the sentences for the type of validity or reliability discussed. (Terms may be used more than once.)

Content   Test-retest
Factor analysis   Cronbach's alpha
Convergent   Alternate or parallel form
Divergent   Interrater
Concurrent

1.   In tests for reliability, the self-efficacy scale had a(n) _____ of 0.88, demonstrating internal consistency for the new measure.

2.   The ABC social support scale demonstrated _____ validity with correlation of 0.84 with the XYZ interpersonal relationships scale.

3.   _____ validity was supported with a correlation of 0.42 between the ABC social support scale and the QRS loneliness scale.

4.   The investigator established _____ validity through evaluation of the cardiac recovery scale by a panel of cardiac clinical nurse specialists. All items were rated 0 to 5 for importance to recovery and only items scoring above an average of 3 were kept in the final scale.

5.   The results of the _____ were that all the items clustered around three factors, lending support to the notion that there are three dimensions of coping.

6.   The observations were rated by three experts. The _____ reliability among the observers was 94%.

7. To assess _____ reliability, subjects completed the locus of control questionnaire at the beginning of the project and 2 weeks later. The correlation of 0.86 supports the stability of the concept.

8. The Heart Health and Recovery Test (HHRT) was developed by the interdisciplinary heart health group. They established _____ validity by reviewing the literature reviewing concerns identified by patients recovering from a cardiac event, and had the items critiqued by a panel of experts.

9. The results of the HHRT that measured threat were highly correlated with the results of a test measuring negative emotions. This established _____ validity.

10. The interdisciplinary heart health study group reported that internal consistency reliabilities of the five factors of the HHRT were computed with the _____ statistic.

REFERENCES

Alhusen, J. L., Gross, D., Hayat, M. J., et al. (2012). The influence of maternal-fetal attachment and health practices on neonatal outcome in low-income, urban women. *Research in Nursing & Health, 35,* 112-120.

Melvin, K. C., Gross, D., Hayat, M. J., et al. (2012). Couple functioning and post-traumatic stress symptoms in US Army couples: The role of resilience. *Research in Nursing & Health, 35,* 164-177.

Thomas, M. L., Elliott, J. E., Rao, S. M., et al. (2012). A randomized clinical trial of education or motivational interviewing based coaching compared to usual care to improve cancer pain management. *Oncology Nursing Forum, 39*(1), 39-49.

US National Library of Medicine. National Institutes of Health. (January 10, 2013). Retrieved from http://www.ncbi.nlm.nih.gov/pubmed.

Data Analysis:
Descriptive and Inferential Statistics

INTRODUCTION

Measurement is critical to any study. The practitioner is interested in the similarity between the measurements used in a study and those usually found in his or her practice. The researcher thinks about how to measure relevant variables while reading the literature and thinking through the theoretical rationale for the study. Both the practitioner and the researcher wonder about how much faith they can put in the measurements reported.

Practitioners and researchers know that the perfect set of measurements does not exist. The researcher's task is to clearly define the variables, choose accurate measurement tools, and clearly explain how the statistical tools were used. Your task as a practitioner who critically reads research is to consider the researcher's explanation of how and why specific descriptive and inferential statistics were used and ask, "What do these numbers tell me?"

Descriptive statistics are valuable for summarizing data and allowing us to look at salient features about a group of data, but practitioners usually want more information. They want to be able to read about an intervention used with a specific group of individuals and consider the usefulness of that intervention with the patients in their care. The use of inferential statistics provides a way for practitioners to look at the data in a study and decide how easily the results can be generalized to the patients they see on a daily basis.

Initially, numbers tend to be intimidating. The best way to eliminate this source of intimidation is to jump in and play with the numbers. Keep reminding yourself that you have the intelligence and skills to do this. Use the mantras of "I think I can. I think I can," and "Practice, practice, practice," and you will have data analysis mastered. Also keep in mind that this is a lifelong learning process. There will still be times when you read a study with a new twist to the use of a statistical procedure, and back you'll go to the reference books, or pick up the phone to call a colleague.

This chapter is designed to help you with the skills part of the task. First, the exercises in this chapter will provide you with some practice in working with the concept of measurement. Second, you will have the opportunity to think through some of the decisions relevant to the use of descriptive and inferential statistics. The bulk of your effort will be spent digesting data from the studies included in the text.

LEARNING OUTCOMES

On completion of this chapter, you should be able to do the following:

- Differentiate between descriptive and inferential statistics.
- State the purposes of descriptive statistics.
- Identify the levels of measurement in a research study.
- Describe a frequency distribution.
- List measures of central tendency and their use.
- List measures of variability and their use.
- Identify the purpose of inferential statistics.
- Explain the concept of probability as it applies to the analysis of sample data.
- Distinguish between a type I and type II error and its effect on a study's outcome.
- Distinguish between parametric and nonparametric tests.
- List some commonly used statistical tests and their purposes.
- Critically appraise the statistics used in published research studies.
- Evaluate the strength and quality of the evidence provided by the findings of a research study and determine their applicability to practice.

Activity 1

Before you start any of the activities for Chapter 16, make life easier for yourself—create tools that will provide a shortcut. Create a set of reference cards that can also serve as flashcards.

Create your own set of "statistical assistants." Once the cards are finished, carry them with you to the library, or set them on the desk while working on the Internet. Use them when reading research reports. Before long, you will be able to read a piece of research without referring to the stack of statistical assistants, and you will master the best shortcut of all: memorizing the statistical notation. Flipping through the pages of a book looking for a statistical symbol before you can evaluate the use of the statistic will no longer be required.

Gather the following supplies: package of 3 × 5 index cards, preferably lined on one side; pens or a combination of pens and highlighters with different colors; one broad-tipped, black-ink marker, your textbook turned to Chapter 16, Tables 16-1, 16-3, and 16-4.

1. Make three key cards first. On one of the 3 × 5 cards, on the side without lines, use the broad-tipped, black marker and write "INFERENTIAL STATISTICAL TECHNIQUES—relationship" and on another write "INFERENTIAL STATISTICAL TECHNIQUES—difference." Take the third 3 × 5 card and write "DESCRIPTIVE TECHNIQUES" on the unlined side.

2. Turn the *inferential statistics—relationship* card over to the lined side. With one of the colored pens, write on the left side of the card the following list:

   2 variables; interval measure
   2 variables; nominal or ordinal
   >2 variables; interval measure
   >2 variables; nominal or ordinal

   Next to the descriptors at the left, write the tests used for each type of data.

3. Turn the *inferential statistics—difference* card over to the lined side. With one of the colored pens, write on the left side of the card the following list:

    2 groups; interval measure
    2 groups; nominal or ordinal
    1 group; interval measure
    1 group; nominal or ordinal

    Next to the descriptors at the left, write the tests used for each type of data.

4. Do the same with the *descriptive statistics* card. Write on the left side of the card the following list:

    nominal measurement
    ordinal measurement
    interval measurement
    ratio measurement

    Next to the descriptors at the left, write the tests used for each type of data.

5. Each line of the key card should be in a different color. Next, create a stack of statistical assistants.

6. Take a blank card. On the front of each card (unlined side) write the full name of one of the statistical tools using the broad-tipped, black marker (or whatever marker was used to write on the front of the key card) (Example: *mean).*

7. Turn the card over and write the information that corresponds to the appropriate category on the key card on the appropriate line using the appropriate color. If you need assistance with choosing the appropriate information to put on each line, refer to Tables 16-1, 16-3, 16-4; the descriptions of each test in your textbook; and the Critical Thinking Decision Path in Chapter 16 of the text. For example, the lined side of the "mean" would read as follows:

    Mathematical average of all scores
    Interval or ratio data
    Most-used measure of central tendency, often used in tests of significance
    Affected by every score, extreme scores can lead to big changes
    Symbol: (see text)
    Best point for summarizing interval or ratio data

8. These cards will fit into an envelope or any of the small plastic cases that can be purchased from the local bookstore. They will slip into a bookbag, briefcase, or backpack with ease.

Activity 2

Match the level of measurement found in Column B with the appropriate example(s) in Column A. (The levels of measurement in Column B will be used more than once. Table 16-1 from the text can assist you.)

Column A	**Column B**
1. _____ Amount of emesis	a. Nominal
2. _____ Scores on the ACT, SAT, or the GRE	b. Ordinal
3. _____ Height or weight	c. Interval
4. _____ Gender	d. Ratio
5. _____ Satisfaction with nursing care	
6. _____ Use or nonuse of contraception	
7. _____ Class ranking	
8. _____ Number of feet or meters walked	
9. _____ Blood type	
10. _____ Body temperature measured with centigrade thermometer	
11. _____ Body temperature measured with Kelvin thermometer	

Activity 3

If you have taken a course in statistics, you are familiar with the statistical notation used to refer to specific types of descriptive statistics. This activity will serve as a quick review. If you have not yet taken a statistics course, this exercise will provide you with enough information to recognize some of the statistical notations.

This is a *reverse* crossword puzzle; therefore, the puzzle is already completed. Your task is to identify the appropriate clue for each answer found in the puzzle. List the correct clue answers in the spaces provided following the puzzle and clues.

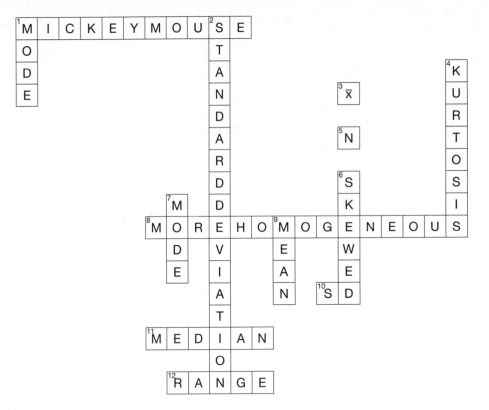

Clues

a. Measure of central tendency used with interval or ratio data
b. Abbreviation for the number of measures in a given data set (the measures may be individual people or some smaller piece of data like blood pressure readings)
c. Measure of variation that shows the lowest and highest number in a set
d. Can describe the height of a distribution
e. Old abbreviation for the mean
f. Marks the "score" where 50% of the scores are higher and 50% are lower
g. Describes a distribution characterized by a tail
h. Abbreviation for standard deviation
i. 68% of the values in a normal distribution fall between +1 of this statistic
j. Goofy's best friend
k. Very unstable
l. The values that occur most frequently in a data set
m. Describes a set of data with a standard deviation of 3 when compared to a set of data with a standard deviation of 12

Across	Down
1.	1.
3.	2.
5.	4.
8.	6.
10.	7.
11.	9.
12.	

Activity 4

Read the following excerpts from specific studies included in your textbook. Identify both the independent and dependent variable(s) and indicate what level of measurement would apply. You may find the Critical Thinking Decision Path in the textbook to be helpful in answering these questions.

1. "Small for gestational age (SGA) was calculated using comprehensive reference values of birth weight at 22-44 completed weeks of gestation that were established by Okenn et al. (2003) based on a national sample of over 6 million infants. The presence of LBW (<2,500G), pre-term birth (<37 completed weeks gestation), or SGA (<10th percentile weight adjusted for gestational age) was coded as an adverse neonatal outcome during data collection. Neonatal outcomes were dichotomized as adverse outcome or no adverse outcome; therefore, multiple logistic regression was used to test the relationships between MFA, health practices, and neonatal outcomes." (Alhusen et al., 2012)

    a. Name the variable of interest.

    b. Identify the level of measurement of this variable.

2. "In univariate logistic regression, MFA was regressed on adverse neonatal outcome and MFA was significantly related to adverse neonatal outcome; the odds ratio for this equation indicated that a one-point increase in MFA was associated with a 9% decreased likelihood of an adverse neonatal outcome." (Alhusen et al. 2012)

    a. Name the independent variable(s).

    b. Name the dependent variable(s).

    c. Identify the level of measurement of the independent variable.

3. "First, the data were explored for gender differences by individual respondents as previously discussed (Table 2). Because this initial analysis did not address the presence or absence of clinical levels of distress, all respondents were then sorted into high or low scores for couple functioning, resilience, and PTSS, based on the clinical cut point of 30. To examine the couples as dyadic units, respondent couples were then sorted into groups based on their scores. Two couple adjustment groups were created: (a) both male and female having high couple adjustment (RDAS scores) and (b) at least one spouse reporting low couple adjustment (RDAS score <48). Similarly, couple groups were created for high and low levels of coercion, using WEB scores >20 in one or more spouses to delineate the abused versus nonabused groups and for PTSS, using PCL scores >30 (see Table 3). Chi-square analysis was used to examine group membership relationships; the results showed there were no significant differences between male and dual military couples on the likelihood of reporting lower couple functioning, higher coercion, or higher PTSS." (Melvin et al., 2012)

    a. What is a dyad? Why do the authors address this concept?

    b. What level of measurement does a researcher need in order to use a chi-square test? What does this test measure?

Activity 5

Use the list of terms to complete the items in this activity. (Some terms may be used more than once.)

ANOVA	Correlation	Nonparametric statistics
Null hypothesis	Parameter	Parametric statistics
Practical significance	Probability	Research hypothesis
Sampling error	Statistic	Statistical significance
Type I error	Type II error	

1. The _____ states that there is no difference between the groups in the study or no association between the variables under study. Its usefulness to a study is that it is the only relationship that can be tested through the use of statistical tools.

2. ANOVA is an example of the use of _____.

3. It is impossible to prove that the _____ is true.

4. The tendency for statistics to fluctuate from one sample to another is known as the _____.

5. The term _____ refers to a characteristic of the population, while the term _____ refers to a characteristic of a sample drawn from a population.

6. When investigators are studying the association between variables, they often will use statistics that measure _____.

7. _____ occurs when the investigator does not find statistical significance but a real difference exists in the world. A(n) _____ occurs when the investigator concludes that there is a real (statistically significant) difference but, in reality, there is no difference.

8. The relative frequency of an event in repeated trials under similar conditions is known as _____ and provides the theoretical basis for inferential statistics.

9. A statistically significant finding based on a change of 3 mm Hg in systolic blood pressure in a sample of healthy individuals likely would have little _____.

10. _____ refer(s) to those tools used when data are collected at the ordinal or nominal level of measurement.

11. When a finding is tested and found to be unlikely to have happened by chance, the investigators report _____ for that particular finding.

12. When a probability level is calculated as $p < 0.05$ and the investigator had set the alpha level of significance at 0.05, the investigator must reject the _____ and accept the _____.

13. Identify the components of the following statistical test result: X^2 (6, $n=213$) = 33.0, $p < .0001$. Match the component with its correct name.

_____ X^2 a. Sample size

_____ 6   b. Degrees of freedom

_____ $n = 213$ c. Chi-square symbol

_____ 33.0   d. Probability level

_____ $p < .0001$ e. Chi-square test statistic

Activity 6

The data in this table contains information from a hypothetical study. Use the statistical assistant cards you developed in Activity 1 to answer the questions that follow.

Table 1
Demographic data ($n = 12$)

Participant	Age	Gender	Income	Antithyroid antibody status	Other autoimmune diseases	Years since thyroid disorder diagnosis
1	27	Female	0+	+	No	3
2	50	Female	$20,001+	−	No	9
3	43	Female	$60,001+	+	Addison's disease	2
4	32	Female	$20,001+	+	No	1
5	66	Male	0+	−	No	14
6	51	Female	$30,001+	+	Rheumatoid arthritis	11
7	78	Female	0+	+	Multiple sclerosis	22
8	missing	Female	missing	+	No	missing
9	44	Female	$40,001+	+	No	8
10	53	Female	$30,001+	+	Rheumatoid arthritis	6
11	32	Male	0+	+	No	3
12	58	Male	missing	−	No	5

1. How big is the sample size?

2. What levels of measurement are represented by the data in this table?

3. For the data in the last column, Years since thyroid disorder diagnosis, what is the mean?

4. For the data in the last column, Years since thyroid disorder diagnosis, what is the median?

5. For the data in the last column, Years since thyroid disorder diagnosis, what is the mode?

6. What is a limitation of using the mean to describe this sample?

Activity 7

Using the studies in Appendices A through D in the textbook, answer the following questions regarding the use of descriptive and inferential statistics in each study. Once again, use Tables 16-3 and 16-4 and Figures 16-2 and 16-3 of the textbook.

1. Were descriptive statistics used in the study?

    a. Thomas et al.

    b. Alhusen et al.

    c. Seiler & Moss

    d. Melvin et al.

2. What data were summarized and/or explained through the use of the descriptive statistics described in your textbook?

    a. Thomas et al.

    b. Alhusen et al.

    c. Seiler & Moss

    d. Melvin et al.

3. Were the descriptive statistics used appropriately?

    a. Thomas et al.

    b. Alhusen et al.

    c. Seiler & Moss

    d. Melvin et al.

4. Did any of the four studies rely more heavily on the use of descriptive statistics than the others? If so, why do you think this occurred?

5. Now turn to the inferential statistics. Which of the four studies in the appendices used some type of inferential statistic to manage the data?

   a. Thomas et al.

   b. Alhusen et al.

   c. Seiler & Moss

   d. Melvin et al.

6. What inferential statistical tools described by your textbook were used in the studies?

   a. Thomas et al.

   b. Alhusen et al.

   c. Seiler & Moss

   d. Melvin et al.

Activity 8: Web-Based Activity

1. Visit wwwdontshake.org. Near the top left of the webpage, click on the "All about SBS/ AHT" tab. Scroll down and click on "SBS statistics" on the left column. Choose the "Scotland Study."

   a. A 95% confidence interval (95% CI) is an indicator of the reliability of the estimate. It is the interval of values that is likely (in this case 95% likely) to contain the unknown population parameter. While it is possible that the true value lies outside this estimate, we have some confidence that it is within these bounds. There are several 95% CI given in this report. Based on what you know about confidence levels and your reading about measures of variability, what can you say about the differences in the confidence intervals?

   b. What are some other statistics used in this report?

Activity 9: Evidence-Based Practice Activity

Evidence-based practice means that you base practice decisions on the best evidence available. In the ideal world, this means practitioners would have a stack of experimental studies with clear conclusions that have direct relevance to an immediate clinical concern. Obviously, this is seldom the case. We use our brains and the best practice information available, and intervene and evaluate.

Assume that the shaken baby statistics from Activity 8 have been consistently reported across several studies of varying designs and sample sizes. What, if any, implications would exist for RNs working in pediatrics or labor and delivery?

POSTTEST

1. Two outpatient clinics measured patient waiting time as one indicator of effectiveness. The mean and standard deviation of waiting time in minutes is reported below. Which outpatient clinic would you prefer, assuming that all other things are equal? Explain your answer.

	Clinic 1	Clinic 2
Mean (in minutes)	40	25
Standard deviation (in minutes)	10	45

2. You are responsible for ordering a new supply of hospital gowns for your unit. Which measure of central tendency would be the most useful in your decision-making? Explain your answer.

3. Matching exercise for measures of central tendency: Draw a line connecting the measure of central tendency with the correct description.

Mode   Most frequent score

Median   Arithmetical average, most stable

Mean   Middle score

Fill in the blanks for the following statements.

4. A _____ distribution is said to have _____ or _____ skew.

5. We use inferential statistics to test a(n) _____.

6. _____ _____ like the normal curve are the basis for all _____ statistics.

7. The _____ _____ states that there is no relationship between the variables.

8. If a researcher accepts a null hypothesis that is *not* true, this is a(n) _____ _____ error.

9. A statistical test for differences in proportions is the _____ _____ test.

REFERENCES

Alhusen, J. L., Gross, D., Hayat, M. J., et al. (2012). The influence of maternal-fetal attachment and health practices on neonatal outcome in low-income, urban women. *Research in Nursing & Health, 35,* 112-120.

Melvin, K. C., Gross, D., Hayat, M. J., et al. (2012). Couple functioning and post-traumatic stress symptoms in US Army couples: The role of resilience. *Research in Nursing & Health, 35,* 164-177.

National Center on Shaken Baby Syndrome. (February 15, 2013). Retrieved from www.dont-shake.org.

Seiler, A., & Moss, V. A. (2012). The experiences of nurse practitioners providing health care to the homeless. *Journal of the American Academy of Nurse Practitioners, 24,* 303-312.

Thomas, M. L., Elliott, J. E., Rao, S. M., et al. (2012). A randomized clinical trial of education or motivational interviewing based coaching compared to usual care to improve cancer pain management. *Oncology Nursing Forum, 39*(1), 39-49.

17

Understanding Research Findings

INTRODUCTION

As the last sections of a research report, the Results and Conclusions sections answer the question "So what?" In other words, it is in these two sections that the investigator "makes sense" of the research, critically synthesizes the data, ties them to a theoretical framework, and builds on a body of knowledge. These two sections are a very important part of the research report because they describe the generalizability of the findings and offer recommendations for further research. Well-written, clear, and concise Results and Conclusions sections provide valuable information for nursing practice. Conversely, poorly written Results and Conclusions sections will leave a reader bewildered, confused, and wondering how or if the findings are relevant to nursing.

LEARNING OUTCOMES

On completion of this chapter, you should be able to do the following:

- Discuss the difference between the Results and the Discussion of the Results sections of a research article.
- Identify the format and components of the Results section.
- Determine if both statistically supported and statistically unsupported findings are appropriately discussed.
- Determine whether the results are objectively reported.
- Describe how tables and figures are used in a research report.
- List the criteria of a meaningful table.
- Identify the format and components of the Discussion section.
- Determine the purpose of the Discussion section.
- Discuss the importance of including generalizability and limitations of a study in the report.
- Determine the purpose of including recommendations in the study report.
- Discuss how the strength, quality, and consistency of evidence provided by the findings are related to a study's results, limitations, generalizability, and applicability to practice.

Activity 1

Knowing what information to look for and where to find it in the Results and Discussions sections of a research report will enable you to interpret the research findings and critique research reports. Identify the section in which the following information from the research report may be found. Put an *R* in the blank space if the information would be found in the Results section and a *D* if the information would be found in the Discussion section.

1. _____ Tables/figures to present large amounts of data

2. _____ Limitations of the study

3. _____ Analysis of each question/hypothesis

4. _____ Strength and quality of the evidence

5. _____ Statistical tests used to analyze the data

6. _____ Statistical software program

7. _____ Recommendations for practice and future research

Activity 2

Match the term in Column B with the appropriate definition in Column A.

Column A	Column B
1. _____ Values that quantify the probable value range within which a population parameter is expected to lie	a. Findings
	b. Generalizability
2. _____ Inferences that the data are representative of similar phenomena in a population beyond the study's sample	c. Limitations
	d. Confidence interval
	e. Recommendations
3. _____ The results, conclusions, interpretations, recommendations, and implications for future research and nursing practice of a study	
4. _____ The researchers' suggestions for the study's application to practice, theory, and further research	
5. _____ Threats to a study's internal or external validity	

Activity 3

For questions 1 through 6, answer True (*T*) or False (*F*).

1. _____ Rarely one study should be a recommendation for action.

2. _____ If the results of a study are not supported statistically or are only partially supported, the study is irrelevant and should not have been published.

3. _____ Good tables repeat what the researchers have written in the text.

4. _____ The researchers should respond objectively to the results in the discussion of the findings.

5. _____ All studies have limitations.

6. _____ Statistically significant findings are the sole means for establishing a study's merit.

POSTTEST

The Results and the Discussion of the Results sections are the researcher's opportunity to examine the logic of the hypothesis(es) or researcher question(s) posed, the theoretical framework, the methods, and the analysis of the study. Using the criteria below, critique the Results and Discussion and Conclusions sections of the study by Melvin et al. (2012) found in Appendix D in the text.

1. Are the results of each of the hypotheses presented?

2. Is the information regarding the results concisely and sequentially presented?

3. Are the tests that were used to analyze the data presented?

4. Are the results presented objectively?

5. If tables or figures are used, a) do they supplement and economize the text, b) do they have precise titles and headings, and c) are they not repetitious of the text?

6. Are the results interpreted in light of the hypotheses and theoretical framework and all of the other steps that preceded the results?

7. If the data are supported, does the investigator provide a discussion of how the theoretical framework was supported?

8. How does the investigator attempt to identify the study's weaknesses—that is, threats to internal and external validity—and strengths, as well as suggest possible solutions for the research area?

9. Does the researcher discuss the study's clinical relevance?

10. Are any generalizations made, and if so, are they within the scope of the findings or beyond the findings?

11. Are any recommendations for future research stated or implied?

REFERENCE

Melvin, K. C., Gross, D., Hayat, M. J., et al. (2012). Couple functioning and post-traumatic stress symptoms in US Army couples: The role of resilience. *Research in Nursing & Health, 35,* 164-177.

Appraising Quantitative Research

INTRODUCTION

Chapter 18 in the textbook includes two thorough critiques of two quantitative studies. The first study critiqued is one by Sherman et al. (2012) that examined the effectiveness of interventions (psychoeducation or psychoeducation plus telephone counseling) for promoting the physical, emotional, and social adjustment of women with early stage breast cancer. The second critique is of a study by Cerdan et al. (2012) that examined the effect of asthma severity on caregivers' quality of life. Critiquing criteria that were presented in all previous chapters were combined and used. The results in Chapter 18 are complete critiques of two separate studies.

Both of these critiques reflect the level of analysis desired for an article that the registered nurse had decided was relevant to practice. If you want to produce a critique at this level of thoroughness, it will take time. It would not be uncommon for a novice reader of research to use two to three hours (maybe more) to complete such a critique. Usually novice readers of research find the task tedious and, not infrequently, difficult. The more often you read and critique studies in this manner, the easier (and more interesting) reading research becomes. The easier it becomes, the more quickly you can complete a critique. To get started, you just have to pick an article, dive in, and do it.

One way of getting started is to commit to work to improve your critiquing skills. For example, you could commit to finding one research study every week that is relevant to an area of nursing you are interested in or a question you have related to nursing practice and critique that article using the steps outlined in the textbook. At the end of a year, you could have read almost four dozen studies.

As mentioned earlier, the level of reading and critiquing is most often used when you have a reasonable expectation that a specific study will be useful in your professional practice. But not all relevant articles will be found in the journals that are devoted specifically to your area of clinical expertise. Often you may find yourself searching through several electronic databases or numerous journals to find studies that can be useful. When you do find a study that appears to be practice-relevant, you need to assess the article quickly so you can decide whether you should be spending the time to critically appraise the study.

LEARNING OUTCOMES

On completion of this chapter, you should be able to do the following:

- Identify the purpose of the critical appraisal process.
- Describe the criteria for each step of the critical appraisal process.
- Describe the strengths and weaknesses of a research report.
- Assess the strength, quality, and consistency of evidence provided by a quantitative research report.
- Discuss applicability of the findings of a research report for evidence-based nursing practice.
- Conduct a critique of a research report.

Activity 1

This quick reading of articles demands the reader consider the same aspects of a study that you would consider if completing a more detailed critique, but in a more superficial manner. This type of reading is called "inspectional reading" (Adler & Van Doren, 1972). Mastering inspectional reading is essential, but is frequently overlooked in regard to analytical skills. Frequently, professional reading must be squeezed into a small window of available time. Improving your quick reading skills will help you sort through the reading required to maintain and expand your knowledge base.

But what is this inspectional reading? It is the second level in a set of skills described by Adler & Van Doren (1972). The first skill is elementary reading, which is usually accomplished very early in formal education. Level two is inspectional reading. Level three is analytical reading where the reader is trying very hard to understand what the author is attempting to share, and is the level of reading required to produce a critique of a research study. Level four is syntopical reading, which requires intense effort to synthesize ideas from many sources.

Inspectional reading has two components. The first is called "systematic skimming" and the second is called "superficial reading."

Systematic skimming is the first thing anyone should do when approaching a research study. It requires only a few minutes to skim an article—but it may take up to an hour if you are skimming a complete book. Let's assume that you are going to skim a hard copy of a research study.

- Read the title and the abstract.
- Read the biographical information about the authors/researchers.
- Read the Conclusions section.
- Ask yourself the following question: Is the clinical question addressed in the study similar to the clinical question that I have?" Or more specifically, are the components of your PICO or PECO or PS question similar to that of the study? Remember PICO includes the patients/population, intervention, comparison, and outcome(s), PECO includes the patients/population, exposure, comparison, and outcome(s), and PS includes the patients/population and the situation. If your answer is "no," it is likely OK to put this study down and move on to the next study or search for another study. If your answer "unsure" or "yes", proceed to superficial reading of the article.

Superficial reading requires that you read the article from beginning to end without stopping. Try your best not to take notes, not to highlight (hide your highlighter so you won't even be tempted), or use a dictionary to understand words that you do not know. Try not to even stop to think "I wonder what they meant by that?" The key to this step … Just read.

When you have completed the article, take a deep breath and ask yourself these questions:

- What do I remember about the study? The question? The methods? The results? The discussion?
- Was the research design experimental, nonexperimental, or qualitative?
- Where would the study fit in terms of level of evidence?
- Did anything in the study raise any ethical questions?
- Does it fit with my clinical question? If the answer is "no," again it's probably time to move on to the next article. If the answer is "maybe" put it in a "come-back-to-later" stack. If the answer is "yes," proceed to more detailed reading while writing down notes that would be necessary to complete a critical appraisal, such as the two examples found in Chapter 18.

Activity 2

The article by Thomas et al. (2012) in Appendix A of the textbook has been used for several activities throughout this Study Guide. However, it is quite possible that you have not read it completely, at one time, from beginning to end. For this activity, consider the following scenario:

You currently work as a registered nurse in an inpatient adult oncology unit. As part of involvement in your unit's journal club, every other month you are responsible for identifying a research study that is relevant to practice. To help you find a relevant research study, you have been asking your colleagues what they think is the most important issue on the unit for patients. The issue of pain management and control is identified as one of the priority issue areas.

Now, read the study by Thomas et al., practicing the use of systematic skimming and inspectional reading strategies. When you have done so, answer the questions that follow.

Systematic skimming:

- What do you know about the authors/researchers?
- How does the clinical question addressed in the study compare to the clinical question in the scenario?

Superficial reading:

- What do I remember about the study? The question? The methods? The results? The discussion?
- Was the research design experimental, nonexperimental, or qualitative?
- Where would the study fit in terms of level of evidence?
- Did anything in the study raise any ethical questions?
- Does it fit with my clinical question?

Activity 3

Often in practice, nurses are asked to summarize their critical appraisal of a research study within a very short timeframe (i.e., 2 to 3 minutes). Consider the same scenario as in Activity 2 and the study by Thomas et al. (2012) in Appendix A. Keeping in mind that this study has been used for several activities throughout the textbook and Study Guide, review the study in terms of the critical appraisal criteria provided in Chapter 18 of the textbook.

In no more than five sentences, summarize the following for the study by Thomas et al. (2012). (Note: Refer to the "Conclusions/Implications/Recommendations" and "Application to Nursing Practice" sections from the two critical appraisal examples in Chapter 18 as a guide.)

- Population (or sample)
- Type of study; i.e., level of evidence
- Strengths and limitations
- Results (i.e., "Is there a difference between the study groups?"; "Is the difference statistically significant?")
- Applicability to practice

POSTTEST

There is no posttest for this chapter. Enjoy the break!

REFERENCES

Adler, M. J., & Van Doren, C. (1972). *How to Read a Book.* New York: Simon & Schuster.

Thomas, M. L., Elliott, J. E., Rao, S. M., et al. (2012). A randomized clinical trial of education or motivational interviewing based coaching compared to usual care to improve cancer pain management. *Oncology Nursing Forum, 39*(1), 39-49.

19

Strategies and Tools for Developing an Evidence-Based Practice

INTRODUCTION

Maintaining a clinical practice that incorporates new evidence can be challenging. This chapter will assist you in becoming a more efficient and effective reader of the literature by providing you with a few important tools to assist you in determining the merits of a study for your practice and patients.

LEARNING OUTCOMES

After reading this chapter, you should be able to do the following:

- Identify the key elements of a focused clinical question.
- Discuss the use of databases to search the literature.
- Screen a research article for relevance and credibility.
- Critically appraise study results and apply the findings to practice.
- Make clinical decisions based on evidence from the literature combined with clinical expertise and patient preferences.

Activity 1

Using the PICO format to organize a clinical question is helpful to the nurse who is searching for the best-available evidence. In addition to determining major search terms, the PICO format also helps the nurse determine the clinical category to which a research study belongs. Follow the instructions below.

(A) Put the following clinical questions into PICO format. (Note: Depending on the questions being asked, in some studies there may be no "C" or comparison).

(B) Identify which clinical category you would expect the study to belong to.

Therapy (T)
Diagnosis (D)
Prognosis(P)
Causation/Harm (C/H)

1. In older adults, do measures of adiposity and cardiorespiratory fitness predict mortality? (Peters, 2008)

   a. P _____

   _____

   b. I _____

   _____

   c. C _____

   _____

   d. O _____

   _____

   e. Clinical Category: _____

2. Is negative pressure wound therapy (NPWT) using vacuum-assisted closure more effective than advanced moist wound therapy (AMWT) for diabetic foot ulcers? (Sandison, 2008)

   a. P _____

   _____

   b. I _____

   _____

   c. C _____

   _____

   d. O _____

   _____

   e. Clinical Category: _____

3. What is the accuracy of the CRAFFT test in screening for substance abuse among adolescents in a hospital-based clinic? (Jull, 2003)

   a. P _____

   _____

   b. I _____

   _____

   c. C _____

   _____

   d. O _____

   _____

   e. Clinical Category: _____

4. Is there an association between the risk of childhood acute lymphoblastic leukemia and residential exposure to magnetic fields from power lines? (Bryant-Lukosius, 1998)

   a. P _____

   _____

   b. I _____

   _____

   c. C _____

   _____

   d. O _____

   _____

   e. Clinical Category: _____

Activity 2: Web-Based Activity

As mentioned above, determining the clinical category of a research study will help in your search for the best-available evidence. Access the following online bibliographic databases and list the clinical category filters for each database below.

1. CINAHL

2. Medline

3. PubMed (Medline)—click "Limits" on top of home page

4. PubMed (Medline)—click on "Clinical Queries" on left side of home page

5. Based on the clinical category filters for each of the bibliographic databases above, which database do you think would provide you the most efficient search if you were able to identify the clinical category of the PICO question you were searching for?

Activity 3

Match the term in Column B with the appropriate interpretation in Column A.

	Column A	**Column B**
1. _____	Number of adults who need to receive the RTS,S vaccine in order to prevent one adult from being diagnosed with a new malaria infection	a. Continuous variable
2. _____	Risk of a new malaria infection being 0.96 times less for adults who receive the RTS,S vaccine than in those who do not receive the RTS,S vaccine	b. Discrete variable
3. _____	Rapid screening tests being 96% accurate in detecting the proportion of patients with a negative test as not having malaria	c. Relative risk
4. _____	Number of patients diagnosed with malaria	d. Relative risk reduction
5. _____	Malaria being 4.8 times more likely to be reported among Swedish children ages 1-6 years than other age groups	e. Odds ratio
6. _____	78% of patients presenting to an outpatient clinic with a positive rapid screening test having malaria	f. Absolute risk reduction
7. _____	Percentage of patients diagnosed with malaria	g. Number-needed-to-treat
8. _____	1% of adults who receive the RTS,S vaccine do not develop a new malaria infection	h. Sensitivity
9. _____	Rapid screening tests being 95% accurate in detecting the proportion of patients with positive tests as having malaria	i. Specificity
10. _____	95% of patients presenting to an outpatient clinic with a negative rapid screening test will not have malaria	j. Positive predictive value
11. _____	RTS,S vaccination reduces new malaria infections by 4% relative to not receiving the vaccination	k. Negative predictive value

Activity 4

As an RN working in an inpatient adult cardiac unit, you are concerned with the effectiveness of pressure bandages applied following angiography procedures. Because you find that the pressure bandages often reduce the patients' mobility and increase patients' reports of discomfort, you perform a literature review to see if pressure bandages are effective for reducing bleeding. You retrieve the randomized controlled trial by Botti et al. (1998). The following is a summary of the design and findings (Donahue, 1999). Use this information to answer the questions below.

Setting: 1 private and 2 public university hospitals in Melbourne, Australia.

Sample: n = 1,705 patients whose average age was 61.4 years, 69% male

Methods: Randomization was stratified across the 3 hospitals. After the coronary angiography procedure was completed and once hemostasis was achieved through >10 minutes of manual compression, patients were allocated to the study groups.

Intervention: Pressure bandage (8 gauze squares held in place by 2-meter elasticized non-adhesive bandage applied in a figure-8 formation around the leg and across the lower abdomen and back, which remained in place for 6-12 hours.

Control: Adhesive bandage or no covering

Findings: 3.5% of patients in the intervention group and 6.7% of patients in the control group experienced bleeding. The RR was 0.52 with 95% CI (0.3, 0.9) and the NNT was 32.

1. How was the outcome variable measured? Was it measured as a continuous or discrete variable?

2. What is the null value of the outcome measure used to interpret the CI?

3. How would you interpret the CI?

4. The results of the study are expressed as an RR. Interpret the RR and determine if it is statistically significant.

5. Interpret the NNT. How was it calculated? Is the NNT clinically useful?

6. How would you apply the results of this study to the clinical situation?

Activity 5

You are volunteering with a school nurse at a local high school in San Francisco, California. In your first few weeks of volunteering, you start to wonder why it seems that most of the teenage girls being diagnosed with eating disorders are those whose parents are divorced. Out of curiosity, you perform a quick literature review to see if the evidence supports your observations. You retrieve the cohort study by Martínez-González et al. (2003). The following is a summary of the design and findings (Newton, 2003). Use this information to answer the questions below.

Setting: Navarra, Spain

Sample: $n = 2{,}862$ girls ages 12-21 years old (mean age 15.5 years old)

Outcomes: Parents' marital status (other versus married); eating alone (yes versus no); reading girls' magazines ($<$ weekly versus $\geq$ weekly); and listening to radio ($\leq$ 1 hour per day versus $>$ 1 hour per day)

Findings: When odds ratios (CI 95%) were adjusted for all variables as well as age, body mass index, self-esteem, and socioeconomic status, of the girls who were clinically diagnosed with eating disorders ($n = 90$), findings indicated that the OR for parents' marital status was 1.97 (1.10 to 3.51), for eating alone was 2.94 (1.88 to 4.60), for reading girls' magazines was 1.42 (0.91 to 2.2), and for listening to radio was 1.55 (1.01 to 2.40).

1. What was the PICO question addressed in the clinical situation?

2. The question addressed in the study by Peterson et al. (2008) was, "Are parental, mass media, sociodemographic, and psychosocial variables associated with an increased risk of developing an eating disorder (ED) in girls?" (Newton, 2003, p. 120). How does the PICO question in the clinical situation compare to the PICO question asked by Peterson et al. (2008)?

3. Based on the PICO question of the clinical situation and the question addressed in the study by Peterson et al. (2008), what clinical category is being addressed? Structured tools are available to help you systematically appraise the strength and quality of evidence for a given category of a clinical question. Although many tools exist, the tools developed by the Critical Appraisal Skills Programme (CASP) are easily accessible and user-friendly to complete. Go to the CASP website (www.phru.nhs.uk/pages/PHD/resources.htm) to determine which of the tools to use to critique the study by Peterson et al. (2008).

4. Indicate whether each of the outcomes are continuous variables (*C*) or discrete variables (*D*).

   a. _____ Parents' marital status

   b. _____ Eating alone

   c. _____ Reading girls' magazines

   d. _____ Listening to radio

5. Interpret the study findings. Which findings are statistically significant? How can you tell?

6. How would you apply the results of this study to the clinical situation? Do the results warrant an evidence-based practice change?

Activity 6: Web-Based Activity

Retrieve and review the following:

Bassler, D., Busse, J. W., Karanicolas, P. J., & Guyatt, G. H. (2008). Evidence-based practice targets the individual patient. Part 1: How clinicians can use study results to determine optimal individual care. *Evidence-Based Nursing, 11*, 103-104.

DiCenso, A. (2001). Clinically useful measures of the effects of treatment. *Evidence-Based Nursing, 4*, 36-39.

POSTTEST

Determine whether each of the following statements is True (*T*) or False (*F*). If an item is False, revise it to make it a True statement.

1. _____ An experimental or quasi-experimental study design is usually used for the causation/harm category of clinical concern used by clinicians.

2. _____ Articles should be screened to determine if the setting and sample in the study are similar to my clinical situation.

3. _____ A confidence interval can provide the reader information about the statistical significance of the findings.

4. _____ *Specificity* is the term used to describe the proportion of individuals with a disease who test positive for it.

5. _____ A confidence interval does not provide the reader information about the clinical significance of the findings.

6. _____ The null value for continuous variables is "0."

7. _____ NNT is a useful measure for applying research findings to practice.

8. _____ *Prevalence* is a term used to describe the number that expresses the sensitivity, specificity, PPV, and NPV.

REFERENCES

Askling, H. H., Nilsson, J., Tegnell, A., Janzon, R., & Ekdahl, K. (2005). Malaria risk in travelers. *Emerging Infectious Diseases, 11*(3), 436-441.

Bassler, D., Busse, J. W., Karanicolas, P. J., & Guyatt, G. H. (2008). Evidence-based practice targets the individual patient. Part 1: How clinicians can use study results to determine optimal individual care. *Evidence-Based Nursing, 11*, 103-104.

Botti, M., Williamson, B., Steen, K., et al. (1998). The effect of pressure bandaging on complications and comfort in patients undergoing coronary angiography: A multicenter randomized trial. *Heart Lung, 27*, 360-373.

Bryant-Lukosius, D. (1998). Childhood acute lymphoblastic leukaemia was not linked to residential exposure to power line magnetic fields. *Evidence-Based Nursing, 1*, 55.

Ciliska, D., Cullum, N., & Marks, S. (2001). Evaluation of systematic reviews for treatment or prevention interventions. *Evidence-Based Nursing, 4*, 100-104.

DiCenso, A. (2001). Clinically useful measures of the effects of treatment. *Evidence-Based Nursing, 4*, 36-39.

Donahue, M. (1999). Pressure bandages after coronary angiography reduced bleeding, but increased discomfort. *Evidence-Based Nursing, 2*, 84.

Graves, P. M., & Gelband, H. (2009). Vaccines for preventing malaria (blood-stage). *Cochrane Database of Systematic Reviews, 18*(4). DOI: 10.1002/14651858.CD006199.

Jull, A. (2003). The CRAFFT test was accurate for screening substance abuse among adolescent clinic patients. *Evidence-Based Nursing, 6*, 23.

Martínez-González, M. A., Gual, P., Lahortiga, F., et al. (2003). Parental factors, mass media influences, and the onset of eating disorders in a prospective population-based cohort. *Pediatrics, 111*, 315-320.

Newton, M. (2003). Eating alone, parents' marital status, and use of radio and girls' magazines were risk factors for eating disorders. *Evidence-Based Nursing, 6*, 120.

Peters, A. (2008). BMI and cardiorespiratory fitness predicted mortality in older adults. *Evidence-Based Medicine, 13*, 90-91.

Reyburn, H., Mbakilwa, H., Mwangi, R., Mwerinde, O., Olomi, R., Drakely, C., et al. (2007). Rapid diagnostic tests compared with malaria microscopy for guiding outpatient treatment of febrile illness in Tanzania: Randomised trial. *British Medical Journal, 334*, 403.

Sandison, S. (2008). Negative pressure wound therapy promoted healing of diabetic foot ulcers more than advanced moist wound therapy. *Evidence-Based Nursing, 11*, 116.

Developing an Evidence-Based Practice

INTRODUCTION

Engaging in evidence-based practice has become an expected standard in the delivery of health care services. Although there are concentrated efforts on methods to facilitate the translation of research findings into practice, nurses can engage in evidence-based practice through the development, implementation, and evaluation of evidence-based changes in practice. This chapter presents an overview of evidence-based practice, and the process for applying evidence in practice to improve patient outcomes.

LEARNING OUTCOMES

On completion of this chapter, you should be able to do the following:

- Differentiate among conduct of nursing research, research utilization, and evidence-based practice.
- Describe the steps of evidence-based practice.
- Identify barriers to evidence-based practice and strategies to address each.
- Describe strategies for implementing evidence-based practice changes.
- Identify steps for evaluating an evidence-based change in practice.
- Use research findings and other forms of evidence to improve the quality of care.

Activity 1

Although the terms *research utilization* and *evidence-based practice* are often used interchangeably, they are not exactly the same. Answer the following to help you differentiate between the two terms.

1. Describe the difference between *research utilization* and *evidence-based practice*.

2. Identify the three major components of evidence-based practice.

a. _____

b. _____

c. _____

Activity 2

Following are short descriptions of RN activities related to research. Each can be categorized as one of the following.

a. Conduct of research
b. Dissemination of research findings
c. Research utilization
d. Evidence-based practice

Place the letter (a, b, c, d) that best describes each activity in the space provided. (Some letters will be used more than once.)

1. _____ The RN submits an article to his or her health care agency's in-house practice newsletter about the research study he or she participated in.

2. _____ As a member of the health care team, the RN was involved with developing a plan of care for a patient using the findings from one meta-analysis and several research studies.

3. _____ Two RNs are involved with data collection for a study comparing two types of dressings for postoperative incisions.

4. _____ The RN has read about an intervention that will reduce the pain associated with the injection of a particular medication. After reviewing all of the variables, he or she decides that trying the intervention would be a good idea and proceeds to develop an implementation plan.

5. _____ Marie has been working with a faculty member on an independent study project. The two of them have decided to publish the results of their work.

6. _____ A journal club group comprised of RNs, MDs, and NPs have identified a specific clinical question and plan to develop a practice guideline by the end of the year.

Activity 3

Number the following major steps of evidence-based practice in the correct sequence. Use the number "1" for the first step.

a. _____ Choose an approach to assess the quality of the individual research and strength of the body of evidence

b. _____ Select a topic

c. _____ Critique the research

d. _____ Implement the evidence-based change in practice

e. _____ Form a team

f. _____ Evaluate the evidence-based change in practice

g. _____ Identify evidence-based practice recommendations

h. _____ Write the evidence-based practice standard

i. _____ Retrieve the best-available evidence

j. _____ Synthesize the evidence

k. _____ Decide if a change in practice is warranted

Activity 4

Fill in the blanks with the appropriate word(s) from the text.

1. Clinical questions arise from different types of "triggers." _____ triggers are identified by staff through quality improvement, risk surveillance, benchmarking data, financial data, or recurrent clinical problems; whereas _____ triggers are ideas generated when staff read research, listen to scientific papers at research conferences, or encounter evidence-based practice guidelines published by federal agencies or specialty organizations.

2. A team is responsible for the development, implementation, and evaluation of an evidence-based practice project. This team is likely to include _____, who are key individuals who will be affected by the implementation of the evidence-based practice project and who are critical to its successful implementation.

3. Formulating clinical questions assists in the retrieval of relevant research and related literature. PICO is one such effective approach to formulating clinical questions. Identify the four components of this acronym: P _____; I _____; C _____; O _____

Activity 5

Once evidence-based practice recommendations have been developed from the critique and synthesis of the best-available evidence, it is then important to determine if these recommendations should result in an evidence-based change in practice. Indicate *yes (Y)* or *no (N)* as to whether the following should be considered in making this decision. The extent to which:

1. _____ there is consistency in findings across studies/guidelines.

2. _____ the evidence was published in peer-reviewed journals.

3. _____ a significant number of studies/guidelines with sample characteristics similar to those to which the recommendations will be used.

4. _____ the studies support current practice.

5. _____ the authors of the studies and/or guidelines are well-known in their field.

6. _____ feasibility exists for use in practice.

Activity 6

Although a practice change may be evidence-based, its adoption depends on several factors. The answers to the following questions will help identify factors influencing the adoption of an evidence-based practice change.

1. According to Rogers' Diffusion of Innovation model, identify two factors that influence the adoption of evidence-based practice innovations.

   a. _____

   b. _____

2. Match the term in Column B with the appropriate interpretation in Column A.

Column A		Column B
a. _____ Practitioners within the local group setting who are expert clinicians, are passionate about the innovation, are committed to improving quality of care, and have a positive working relationship with other health professionals		1. Audit and feedback 2. Opinion leader 3. Change champion 4. Stakeholders
b. _____ Key individual or group of individuals who will be directly or indirectly affected by the implementation of the evidence-based change in practice		
c. _____ Ongoing auditing of performance indicators, aggregating data into reports, and discussing the findings with practitioners during an evidence-based change in practice		
d. _____ Practitioner who is considered by the local group as being dedicated, competent, and trusted to evaluate new information in the context of group norms		

3. Determine whether each of the following strategies have seemed to have a positive effect on promoting the use of evidence-based practices. Place a "Y" next to those you think have a positive effect and a "N" next to those you do not think have a positive effect on evidence-based practices.

    a. Mass media ____

    b. Change champions ____

    c. Didactic education ____

    d. Opinion leaders ____

Activity 7: Web-Based Activity

Retrieve and review the following:

Graham, I. D., & Harrison, M. B. (2005). Evaluation and adaptation of clinical practice guidelines. *Evidence-Based Nursing, 8,* 68-72.

Grimshaw, J. M., Eccles, M. P., Lavis, J. N., Hill, S. J., & Squires, J. E. (2012). Knowledge translation of research findings. *Implementation Science, 7,* 50. Retrieved from http://www.implementationscience.com/content/pdf/1748-5908-7-50.pdf.

Thomas, L. (1999). Clinical practice guidelines. *Evidence-Based Nursing, 2,* 2.

POSTTEST

Retrieve the article by Poppleton, Moynihan, and Hickey (2003) shown in the reference list. Based on the article, answer the following questions about evidence-based practice change.

1. What was the overall topic of the evidence-based practice guideline(s)?

2. Who were members of the evidence-based practice guideline team?

3. Who, if anyone, would you identify as "stakeholders" in the evidence-based practice guideline team? Is there anyone not represented?

4. Was the best-available evidence retrieved? If so, which strategies were used?

5. What was the approach for grading the quality of the individual evidence and strength of the body of evidence?

6. Was the research evidence (existing clinical practice guidelines, systematic reviews [including meta-analyses and/or meta-syntheses], and primary sources/individual research studies) critiqued?

7. Was the research evidence synthesized? What were the evidence-based practice change recommendations?

8. Was the evidence-based practice change written in detail?

9. How was the decision to make the evidence-based practice change supported?

10. Is a method for evaluating the effectiveness of the evidence-based practice change identified?

11. Was the evidence-based practice change evaluated? Was it successful?

12. What were the strategies used by the evidence-based change team to promote the adoption of the evidence-based practice change?

REFERENCES

Centre for Evidence-Based Healthcare. (September 1, 2009). Evidence-Based Medicine Informatics Project: How to use clinical practice guidelines, 2001. Retrieved from www.cche.net/usersguides/guideline.asp.

Graham, I. D., & Harrison, M. B. (2005). Evaluation and adaptation of clinical practice guidelines. *Evidence-Based Nursing, 8,* 68-72.

Poppleton, V. K., Moynihan, P. J., Hickey, P. A. (2003). Clinical practice guidelines: The Boston experience. *Progress in Pediatric Cardiology, 18,* 75-83.

Thomas, L. (1999). Clinical practice guidelines. *Evidence-Based Nursing, 2,* 2.

Titler, M. G., Mentes, J. C., Rakel, B. A., et al. (1999). From book to bedside: Putting evidence to use in the care of the elderly. *Joint Commission Journal on Quality Improvement, 25*(10), 545-556.

Uribe, S. (2006). Prevention and management of dental decay in the pre-school child. *Evidence-Based Dentistry, 7,* 1.

21

Quality Improvement

INTRODUCTION

We've all had moments as nurses or as patients where we can see how the efficiency of a health care process could improve or how safety could be increased. As nurses, we are on the front lines providing care and we have the tools to affect changes in health care that can make a meaningful difference for our patients. Not every improvement in care is due to a large scientific study and, in fact, many improvements in the quality of care come from small changes based on quality improvement (QI). QI uses data to improve the quality and safety of health care by monitoring outcomes of care processes. QI employs improvement methods to continuously aim for better care by designing and testing changes. QI complements EBP and research efforts to improve care.

Efficiency, access, safety, timeliness, and patient-centeredness problems in clinical settings are ideal candidates for quality improvement solutions. Nurses play key roles in QI activities, and as a nurse you will probably be involved in QI activities in your professional capacity. With a basic understanding of QI, you will be prepared to play your role in improving care for your patients.

LEARNING OUTCOMES

On completion of this chapter, you should be able to do the following:

- Discuss the characteristics of quality health care as defined by the Institute of Medicine.
- Compare the characteristics of the major QI models used in health care.
- Identify two databases used to report health care organizations' performance to promote consumer choice and guide clinical QI activities.
- Describe the relationship between nurse-sensitive quality indicators and patient outcomes.
- Describe the steps in the improvement process and determine appropriate QI tools to use in each phase of the improvement process.
- List four themes for improvement to apply to the unit where you work.
- Describe ways that nurses can lead QI projects in clinical settings.
- Use the SQUIRE guidelines to critique a journal article reporting the results of a QI project.

Activity 1

Quality improvement efforts are one part of the wider effort to improve patient care. QI, evidence-based practice, and research have many similarities that may be confusing. In this exercise, we'll build a table of the major differences in QI, EBP, and research based on what you have learned in Chapter 21 and throughout this textbook. Please fill in each column after reviewing the final chapter in your book.

	Quality Improvement	Evidence-Based Practice	Research
Purpose			
Rigor ←→ control			
Method			
Human subjects			
Data collection			
Results			
Dissemination			

Activity 2

Now that you have thought about the differences between QI, EBP, and research, let's examine some of the similarities. Write a short sentence or two about what you see that is similar among QI, EBP, and research.

1. _____

   _____

2. _____

   _____

3. _____

   _____

4. _____

   _____

5. _____

   _____

Activity 3

Quality improvement follows similar steps to the nursing process. In this exercise you will describe how the QI process steps parallel and differ from the nursing process.

Quality Improvement	Nursing Process
	1. Assessment: collecting, organizing, and analyzing information or data about the patient. Subjective or objective data. Collected by observation, interview, examination. Data are reviewed and interpreted. Develop problem list and prioritize patient's problems.
	2. Nursing diagnosis. Statement that describes and actual or potential problem.
	3. Plan. Devise plan using patient goals and nursing orders to provide care that will meet patient's needs. Set patient goals.
	4. Implement. Carry out the nursing care plan you devised. Reassess the patient. Validate that the care plan is accurate. Implement nursing orders. Document.
	5. Evaluate. Compare patient's current status with stated goals. Were goals achieved? Review nursing process.

Activity 4: Web-Based Activity

1. Go to http://www.medicare.gov/hospitalcompare/search.aspx and search for a hospital you have worked in during your clinical experience or a hospital in your area.

2. Look at the following tabs: "Patient survey results," "Timely and effective care," "Readmissions, complications, and death," and "Use of medical imaging." Do you see any problem areas that need some work?

3. Based on your experience and readings, brainstorm some potential QI solutions to these problem areas.

Activity 5: Evidence-Based Practice Activity

1. Themes for improvement in QI include eliminating waste, improving workflow, optimizing inventory, changing work environments, time management, managing variation, designing systems to avoid mistakes, and focusing on products or services.

2. Think of nursing problems you have encountered in your clinical areas or through your reading. Have you done a literature search on any of these topics?

3. Review the literature you have found, or run a search on a topic of interest to you.

4. Evaluate the top 5 articles according to the critical decision tree in Figure 21-6 in your textbook. Is your article a research study or a QI study? What were the critical clues that helped you decide? Critically think about your new understanding of the differences among QI, EBP, and research. Do you feel that you understand the literature better?

POSTTEST

1. The following are characteristics of quality health care according to the IOM: care that is _____, _____, _____, _____, _____, and _____.

2. _____ is one method for tracking performance and knowing when performance is below the accepted standard and in need of QI.

3. The steps of the QI process are: _____, _____, _____ _____, and _____.

4. A lead QI team should include representatives from the professions involved in patient care, _____, _____, and _____.

5. System variation may be due to random causes or _____ or it may be due to _____.

6. Publication and dissemination of the results of QI studies have been difficult due to the limits on generalizability of this type of work, the _____ guidelines were developed to promote publication of QI studies.

7. *PDSA* stands for _____ _____ _____ _____ , and is part of the _____.

REFERENCE

Medicare Hospital Compare: Quality of Care. (February 21, 2012). Retrieved from www.hospitalcompare.hhs.gov.

Answer Key

CHAPTER 1

Activity 1
1. c
2. d
3. b
4. a
5. g
6. e
7. f
8. h
9. i

Activity 2
1. b
2. b
3. a
4. b
5. a
6. a
7. b

Activity 3
1. Preliminary
2. Comprehensive
3. Parts; whole

Activity 4
1. a. Level IV (cohort study)
   b. Level IV (cross-sectional study)
   c. Level 1 (systematic review with meta-analysis)
2. Answers will vary

Activity 5
1. b
2. a
3. c

Activity 6
1. Introduction
2. Abstract, Introduction
3. Introduction
4. Introduction
5. Introduction
6. Abstract, Introduction
7. Abstract, Methods (Sample & Setting), Results (Sample)
8. Not stated
9. Methods (Instruments)
10. Methods (Instruments)
11. Methods (Procedures)
12. Methods (Data Analysis)
13. Results
14. Discussion
15. Conclusions & Implications for Nursing Practice

POSTTEST
1. a. Concepts: pain, disability
   b. Will vary for each student.
   c. Will vary for each student. Possibilities include the following: How was pain defined, and do you agree with that concept of pain? Does limitation in one item on a scale equal functional disability? How do the patients define functional disability?
2. Both research and evidence-based practice begin with a question.
3. In research, the question is explored with a design appropriate to the question and specific methodology to contribute to new knowledge. In evidence-based practice, the question is used to guide the search for knowledge (research) to address the question.

4. Both qualitative and quantitative research aim to generate new knowledge using designs appropriate to the question being asked.
5. Qualitative research seeks to interpret the meaning of phenomena, whereas quantitative research seeks to test hypotheses using statistical methods to explore phenomena.

CHAPTER 2

Activity 1
1. f
2. b
3. d
4. a
5. c
6. e

Activity 2
1. Yes; Yes; Yes
2. Yes; Yes; No
3. Yes; Yes; Yes
4. Yes; No; Yes
5. Yes; No; Yes

Activity 3
1. a
2. a
3. b
4. a
5. b

Activity 4
1. a. Iron
   b. Iron status
2. a. Family-centered care
   b. Health-related quality of life
3. a. continuous albuterol (usual or high dose)
   b. peak flow
4. a. dental prophylaxes
   b. glycemic control
5. a. parenting
   b. blood pressure and heart rate

Activity 5
1. DH
2. NDH
3. NDH
4. DH
5. DH

Activity 6
1. Yes
2. Yes
3. Yes
4. Yes
5. Yes
6. Yes
7. Yes

Activity 7
1. P = children with long bone fractures in ED
   I = intranasal fentanyl
   C = intravenous morphine
   O = pain control
2. P = obese school-age children and their parents
   I = group intervention
   C = routine care
   O = weight loss
3. P = men after laparoscopic radical prostatectomy
   I = none
   C = none
   O = experiences

POSTTEST
1. The authors state that the purpose of this study was to "test the effectiveness of two interventions compared to usual care in decreasing attitudinal barriers to cancer pain management, decreasing pain intensity, and improving functional status and quality of life" (Melvin et al., 2012).
2. Quantitative
3. a. Yes
   b. Yes
   c. Yes
4. P = Patients diagnosed with cancer experiencing pain with a life expectancy greater than six months; I(1) = motivational interviewing-based coaching; I(2) = education; C = usual care; O = attitudinal barriers to pain management, pain, and quality of life
5. IV = motivational interviewing-based coaching or education; DV = attitudinal barriers to pain management, pain, and quality of life
6. Yes; The article states that "the authors hypothesized motivational interviewing-based coaching group would demonstrate greater benefit (i.e., decreasing attitudinal barriers;

decreasing pain intensity; and improving pain relief, functional status, and quality of life) greater than either the conventional education or usual care groups" (Thomas et al., 2012). It is a directional hypothesis.

CHAPTER 3

Activity 1
1. P
2. S
3. S
4. P

Activity 2
1. PR
2. PR
3. PR
4. NPR
5. NPR
6. PR

Activity 3
1. 124
2. Approximately 540,000
3. CINAHL
4. CINAHL

Activity 4
1. "Studies" and "Syntheses" are found in each of the versions, and include the same type of evidence in each pyramid. Although "Systems" are in each version of the pyramid, in the 4S Pyramid this level includes evidence-based textbooks (i.e., Clinical Evidence, UpToDate) that shift into the "Summaries" level in the 5S and 6S Pyramids. "Summaries" appear in the 5S and are still in the 6S Pyramid, with the same description in both the 5S and 6S. The "Synopses" level in the 4S and 5S Pyramids is broadened to two levels, "Synopses of Syntheses" and "Synopses of Studies" in the 6S Pyramid.

Activity 5
1. Yes. The authors stated the purpose of the study (research questions) and hypotheses in the last paragraph before the "Methods" section begins.
2. Yes. The literature discusses important concepts such as "cancer pain" and "pain

management interventions" and "coaching." The literature review first discusses information about pain management in general and then discusses types of interventions; i.e., psychoeducational and coaching.
3. No
4. Somewhat. The literature review provided details about the types of studies and identifies the limitation of some of the studies; however, the strengths are not identified. There is some discussion of differences between studies. For example, among psychoeducational interventions, those that were less labor-intensive were not as successful in decreasing cancer pain.
5. Yes. Although limited to mostly the findings, the literature review provides a brief summary and provides the references for each research and conceptual article.
6. Yes. "Given the limitations of previous intervention studies, additional research is warranted using approaches that can be implemented in the outpatient setting" (Thomas et al., 2012). In the literature review, the authors discuss that additional studies are needed to test different interventions on cancer pain education. In addition, the authors indicate that psychoeducational interventions may be effective, but they may be considered labor-intensive and not tested in outpatient settings. The authors also indicate that studies have shown that coaching may be a useful strategy to improve cancer pain management.

POSTTEST
1. "Studies", the last level
2. a. P, NPR
   b. P, PR
   c. S, NPR
3. Yes
4. Yes. The authors stated the purpose of the study and hypotheses in the last full paragraph before the "Theoretical Model" section begins.
5. Yes. The literature review provides information about birth rates among low-income and African-American women and then discusses factors known to influence neonatal outcomes (mother's health practices and maternal-fetal attachment).
6. No.

7. No.
8. Yes. Although the findings are limited, the literature review provides a brief summary along with the corresponding references.
9. Yes. The authors state that "No longitudinal studies were found that examine these variables in relation to neonatal outcomes. An enhanced understanding of the role that MFA plays in neonatal outcomes of those subject to disparities, by virtue of race or socioeconomic status, is necessary to improve understanding of the relationship between health practices and adverse neonatal outcomes. Extant literature supports the influence of maternal health practices on neonatal outcomes, but less is known about factors that contribute to a woman's ability to engage in those positive health practices."

CHAPTER 4

Activity 1
1. describe and explain the concept or construct.
2. devise a way to identify and confirm the presence of the concept or construct.
3. determine a method to measure or quantify the concept or construct.

Activity 2
1. e
2. f
3. a
4. b
5. d
6. c

Activity 3
1. Grand; most abstract level of theory
2. Middle range
3. Situation-specific or micro-range; least abstract level of theory

Activity 4
1. Theory is generated as the outcome of a research study.
2. Theory is used as a research framework, as the context for a study.
3. Research is undertaken to test a theory.

Activity 5
a. 3
b. 1
c. 4
d. 2

POSTTEST
1. b, c
2. a
3. c
4. b
5. a
6. a
7. b
8. b
9. f
10. t
11. t
12. f
13. f
14. f
15. t

CHAPTER 5

Activity 1
a. Naturalistic setting: where people live every day; homes, schools, communities.
b. Sample: group of people that the researcher will interview or observe in the process of collecting data to answer the research question.
c. Purposive sample: nonprobability sampling where a researcher selects subjects considered typical of the population.
d. Recruitment: finding and engaging participants in the research.
e. Data saturation: point where enough data have been collected that the information being shared becomes repetitive; no new ideas are emerging.
f. Setting: places where participants are recruited and the data are collected.
g. Themes: overarching, broad categories of meaning.

Activity 2

	Qualitative	Quantitative
Sample Recruitment	Until data saturation	Predetermined number of participants
Data Collection	Naturalistic setting; numbers	Statistics and numbers

Activity 3

Element	Summary
Purpose	"The purpose of this study was to determine the experiences of NPs who provide health care to the homeless in order to gain insight into their unique experience and learn what it takes to be successful in their role" (p. 305)
Method	Qualitative research
Sample and Setting	NPs practicing for at least 6 months in southeast and northeast Wisconsin clinics that provided health care to the homeless
Data Collection	Demographic questionnaire and open-ended interview

POSTTEST

1. a. Quantitative
    b. Qualitative
    c. Qualitative
    d. Qualitative
    e. Quantitative
    f. Qualitative
2. (1) Review of the literature: extensive, systematic, critical review of most important published scholarly literature on the topic
    (2) Study design: blueprint for a study
    (3) Sample: representative units from a population, description of process for selection
    (4) Study setting: description of where subjects were recruited and where data collection occurred
    (5) Data collection: description of how informed consent was obtained, what occurred between contact with the participant and the end of the interview, how were data collected, was a recording made, how long was the interview
    (6) Data analysis: how did the researcher take the raw data—words—and analyze them to find commonalities and differences; usually you will find an example
    (7) Findings: a presentation of the results, a description of the phenomenon, and the role or theme

CHAPTER 6

Activity 1

1. d
2. a
3. c
4. e
5. b
6. f
7. g

Activity 2

1. Identifying the phenomenon	
Phenomenology	Study of day-to-day existence for a particular group of people
Grounded Theory	Interested in social processes from perspective of human interactions or patterns of action and interaction between and among various types of social units
Ethnography	Study of the description and interpretation of a cultural or social groups and systems
Case Study	A focus on an individual, family, community, an organization, or some other complex phenomenon
Community-Based Participatory Research	A study to systematically assess the voice of a community to plan context-appropriate action

2. Structuring the Study	
Phenomenology	Asks about the lived experience, research perspective is bracketed, sample has either lived in the past or is living the experience being investigated.
Grounded Theory	Questions address basic social processes and tend to be action-oriented. The researcher brings some knowledge of the literature but exhaustive review is not done before beginning the research. The sample would be participants who are experiencing the circumstance and selecting events or incidents related to the social processes being studied.
Ethnography	Questions are about lifeways or patterns of behavior within a social context of a culture or subculture. The researcher attempts to make sense of world from insider's point of view. The sample often consists of key informants who have special knowledge, status, or communication skills and who are willing to teach the ethnographer about the phenomenon of interest.
Case Study	Questions about issues that serve as a foundation to uncover complexity and pursue understanding. The perspective of the researcher is reflected in the questions. Researchers may choose the most common cases or instead select the most unusual ones.
Community-Based Participatory Research	Assumes that a phenomenon may be separated from its context. Researchers recognize that engaging members of the study population as active and equal participants, in all phases of research, is crucial.

3. Data Collection

Phenomenology	Written or oral data may be collected.
Grounded Theory	Data are collected through interviews and skilled observations of individuals interacting in a social setting.
Ethnography	Participant observation, immersion, informant interviews
Case Study	Use of interview, observations, document reviews, and other methods
Community-Based Participatory Research	Engage stakeholders in discovering the answers to the community problems

4. Data Analysis

Phenomenology	Move from the participant's description to the researcher's synthesis of all participants' descriptions.
Grounded Theory	Data collection and analysis occur simultaneously, use theoretical sampling, constant comparative method, and axial coding.
Ethnography	Data are collected and analyzed simultaneously, searching for meaning of cultural symbols in the informants' language.
Case Study	Data are often collected and analyzed simultaneously, reflecting and revising meanings.
Community-Based Participatory Research	This stage of research is the "think" phase and is where what has been learned is interpreted or analyzed. The research has the role of linking the ideas provided by the stakeholders in an understandable way so that evidence for specific ways to address the problem can be provided to the community group.

5. Description of the Findings

Phenomenology	A narrative elaboration of the lived experience.
Grounded Theory	Descriptive language and diagrams to show theory connections to the data.
Ethnography	Large quantities of data that provide examples from the data and propositions about relationships of phenomena.
Case Study	Chronologically developed cases, a story that describes case dimensions or vignettes that emphasize various aspects of the case.
Community-Based Participatory Research	Information obtained in earlier research stages sets the stage for community planning, implementation, and evaluation.

Activity 3

1. The article states that the research design used in this study is a "qualitative, naturalistic approach … using the principles of phenomenology."
2. The authors used purposive samples identified through snowball sampling of "NPs practicing for at least 6 months in southeast and northeast Wisconsin clinics that provided health care to the homeless."
3. The procedures are a demographic questionnaire and open-ended interviews. On main question, following by further probing questions were used. Field notes were

collected during the interview and throughout the data collection process. Audiotaped interviews were transcribed verbatim.

4. Data were analyzed using descriptive phenomenology described by Spiegelberger. The researcher read the transcripts while listening to the recordings to immerse in the data. Data were clustered into themes.

Activity 4

1. C
2. B
3. A
4. A
5. B
6. D
7. C
8. A
9. C
10. D
11. C
12. C
13. B
14. A
15. D
16. A (could also be true of B or C)
17. A (could also be true of B or C)
18. C
19. C (could also be true of A)
20. B
21. B

POSTTEST

1. T
2. T
3. F
4. T
5. F
6. a
7. d
8. b
9. a
10. c
11. d
12. a, b, d, or f
13. c

CHAPTER 7

Activity 1

1. g

2. e
3. c
4. f
5. d
6. b
7. h
8. f
9. a
10. g
11. h
12. e

Activity 2

1. Qualitative research provides the opportunity to give voice to those who have been disenfranchised and have no history.
2. Qualitative research creates solutions to practical problems.
3. Qualitative research initiates the examination of important concepts in nursing practice, education, or administration.
4. Qualitative research discovers evidence about a phenomenon of interest that can lead to instrument development.

Activity 3

1. Credibility refers to qualitative research steps taken to ensure the accuracy, validity, and soundness of the data. Credibility can be confirmed when the informants recognize the reported findings as their personal experience.
2. Auditability is a research process that allows the work of a qualitative researcher or a person critiquing a research report to follow the thinking and/or conclusions of a researcher. Auditability can be confirmed when others, not engaged in the research, are able to follow the audit trail of the primary researchers.
3. Fittingness (or transferability) is a term used to answer these three questions: "Are the findings applicable outside the study?", "Are the results or feelings meaningful to people not involved in the research?", and "Are the findings meaningful to others who are in similar situations?" Fittingness is confirmed when the reader is provided with an opportunity to determine the usefulness of the data outside the study.

Activity 4: Web-Based Activity

Your instructor may want to direct you to view some specific Internet links to learn additional specific aspects of qualitative research.

POSTTEST

1. t
2. f
3. t
4. f
5. f
6. d
7. a
8. b
9. c

CHAPTER 8

Activity 1

1. h
2. l
3. e
4. k
5. d
6. j
7. b
8. a
9. c
10. f
11. g
12. i

Activity 2

All of the following are threats to internal validity. Threats to internal validity are alternate explanations of the relationship between the variables and they are potential sources of bias.

1. Testing – The scores on an instrument may improve just from taking the test again, but this effect is hard to distinguish from changes due to the experimental variable. Suggested remedies: Soloman 4 design or use equivalent forms of the instrument.
2. Instrumentation – The differences in variables are due to changes in measurement, not due to the study. Suggested remedies: calibration of study equipment; or for observational data, use similar training for all data collectors.
3. History – Events inside or outside the study have an effect on the dependent variable;

consequently, the effect of these influences is difficult to differentiate from the effect of the independent variable. Suggested remedies: data from some cohorts may be excluded from the analysis; if the whole sample was affected, the author should include this information in the study or may elect to redo the study.

4. Selection Bias – The subjects in a study may not be a representative sample of the population of interest. Suggested remedy: random assignment of subjects to groups.
5. Mortality – Loss of subjects from the study. Suggested remedies: analysis of the subjects who remain in the study and those who dropped out to determine if there was a difference, examination of where the subjects dropped out; for instance, did more subjects drop out of the experimental group than the control group? Researchers may oversample to ensure that they will have an adequate sample even after attrition. They may also use a pilot study to determine if there is a factor in the experimental or control group that may lead to differential loss of subjects.
6. Maturation – A process that operates within an individual as a function of time that is external to the study. Suggested remedy: use a short time interval between the testing periods.

Activity 3

1. The study setting was outpatient oncology clinics including three VA facilities in California, a county hospital in California, a community-based practice in California, and a VA clinic in New Jersey.
2. The subjects were 318 patients with cancer-related pain.
3. A convenience sample was selected by the following method: clinic staff identified and screened potential participants for eligibility and obtained informed consent. Patients were eligible for participation if they were able to read and understand English, had access to a telephone, had a life expectancy greater than 6 months, and had an average pain intensity of 2 or more on a scale from 0-10, where higher scores indicate more pain.
4. Concurrent cognitive or psychiatric condition, substance abuse problem that would prevent adherence to the protocol, severe pain unrelated to their cancer, or residence in

a setting where the patient could not self-administer pain medication.

5. Yes, the groups differed on KPS score but there were no other significant demographic or clinical differences.

6. The Barrier Questionnaire (BQ), to measure attitudinal barriers, the Brief Pain Inventory (BPI) to measure pain, the SF-36 to measure functional status, the FACT-G to measure quality of life. Constancy was maintained by extensive research team training in enrollment, data collection, and interventions. All interventions were standardized across clinic sites. The research associates were also trained in attention-control phone calls. The nurse interventionists were trained in motivational interviewing and change theory by a cognitive behavioral psychologist and in specific procedures related to the coaching protocol. There were also monthly team meetings. Patients and clinicians at the study sites were blinded to the patient's group assignment. Patients in the coaching group received four 30-minute telephone sessions plus the same intervention as the education group. The education group watched a video on managing cancer pain and a written a pamphlet on managing pain. The control group viewed a video on cancer. Patients in the control and education groups received four attention-control phone calls.

7. The usual care group acted as the control.

Activity 4

Your critique may differ from the critique below. Look for similarities in the major points and refer to your textbook if you have questions.

1. Yes, the design is appropriate. The study authors wanted to evaluate the effectiveness of two interventions to decrease attitudinal barriers to cancer-pain management versus usual care and they used a randomized controlled trial to do this.

2. Yes, the methods used for control are consistent with the research design. Control is managed by ruling out extraneous or mediating variables that would compete with the independent variables as an explanation for the study's outcome. Thomas et al. maintain control of extraneous variables by using research team training, written

protocols for nurse interventionist training and coaching interventions, monthly team meetings, consistent data collection procedures, attention-control telephone calls in the usual care and education groups, and randomization of the sample into groups based on stratification by pain intensity and cancer therapy.

3. Time, the study collected data at baseline and again at 6 months: data collection occurred over a long period. Subject availability: the study used outpatient cancer patients. Equipment required included questionnaires, telephones, written materials, video viewing equipment.

4. Yes, the problem ties in nicely with the study framework (the Transtheoretical Model of change theory). The authors provide a solid literature review as a strong basis for the intervention.

5. Threats to internal validity include: history, instrumentation, mortality, and selection bias. The authors also noted that patients in the attention-control call groups reported significant problems during the calls, thereby possibly obscuring some of the effect of the coaching intervention. To reduce the effects of selection bias, participants were stratified and then randomly assigned to groups at each clinic site. To reduce the effects of mortality, the study ended 6 weeks after the coaching intervention, but in hindsight, the investigators would have added another assessment immediately after the end of the coaching intervention to gather data from patients who completed the intervention but were too sick or died before completing the questionnaires.

6. Selection, reactive effects, measurement effects
   a. Selection: sample was comprised mainly of middle-aged, married men
   b. Reactive effects: it is possible that there could have been some positive outcomes simply from being included in the study and receiving phone calls. This possibility was discussed by the authors in relation to the education and usual care groups where some patients used the attention-control phone calls to report significant problems to the research assistant. These problems were then reported to the clinical team (ethically, this was the right

response, but this may have blunted the effect of the coaching intervention).

c. Measurement: instruments that were given at more than one point in time during the study include the BQ, BPI, SF-36, and the FACT-G.

Activity 5

It is possible to ascertain from the titles whether a study was most likely qualitative or quantitative. Results will depend on the year selected. However, this is an excellent site to learn about the most current funded research studies that are taking place. If you find a topic that is of interest to you, you may want to look for an article by the author, or if it is not yet published, you could contact the author as his or her university affiliation is listed.

Activity 6

1. Since your population of interest was not included in the study, you would not include the data from this study in the evidence reviewed for your problem. However, the literature cited by the author in the literature review may be a source of information for your review and should be investigated further.

2. The authors describe nearly all of the potential methods for maintaining constancy. You expect this because it was an intervention study and requires the highest levels of fidelity. The authors may not have described how they knew subjects had understood the intervention prior to the return demonstration, but they tested the subject ability and retested after a period away from the study. You would probably choose to trust that intervention fidelity was maintained if you felt that the steps taken, and described, in the report were adequate.

3. Yes. A negative finding in your area is just as important as a positive finding. Your critiquing criteria would assess validity of the study, any potential weaknesses would be noted, and the results would be included in your evidence.

4. Yes. You would likely need help from a librarian to develop a literature search to identify populations similar to your population. You would decide if the included studies were clinically relevant to your population.

POSTTEST

1. a. Purpose: To examine relationships between maternal-fetal attachment, health practices during pregnancy (rest/exercise, safety, nutrition, avoiding harmful substances, obtaining health care, and obtaining information), and neonatal outcomes (gestational age, birthweight) in a sample of African-American pregnant women reporting low educational attainment and low SES.

   b. Rubin's (1967) theory of maternal role attainment (MRA) and Mercer's expansion of the MRA, the "Becoming a Mother" (BAM) (2004) theory.

   c. Poor (>95% receiving Medicaid), African-American (>95% from the inner city) in the Mid-Atlantic region, >16 years old, between 24-28 weeks gestation with a singleton pregnancy, able to speak English.

   d. Previous treatment with tocolytic therapy, diagnosed preeclampsia or gestational diabetes, diagnosed with a chronic medical condition, abnormal diagnostic result during the current pregnancy, history of spontaneous fetal or infant death.

   e. Maternal-Fetal Attachment Scale (MFAS), Health Practices in Pregnancy Questionnaire II (HPQ-II), pregnancy outcomes (electronic chart review), demographic and pregnancy information.

   f. The authors controlled for income, pregnancy wantedness, preeclampsia, and gestational diabetes through their inclusion/exclusion criteria and during statistical analyses.

2. a. Control
   b. Constancy
   c. External validity
   d. Maturation
   e. Feasibility
   f. Internal validity
   g. Selection bias

CHAPTER 9

Activity 1

1. Experimental
2. Solomon four-group

3. Time series
4. After-only
5. After-only nonequivalent control group
6. True experimental
7. Nonequivalent control group

Activity 2

1. Yes, this study used a true experimental design. This study had random assignment to groups and the group assignment was concealed. There were several processes used to maintain control: manipulation of the independent variable, random assignment to group, use of a control group, preparation of intervention and data collection protocols. Finally, the study also had manipulation, whereby different types of treatment were compared.

2. An experimental design is the best way to test cause and effect since it allows the researcher to eliminate threats to internal validity. They must meet the following conditions to infer causality: The independent and dependent variables must be associated, the cause must precede the effect, and the relationship must not be explained by another variable.

3. a. The independent variables include: motivational interviewing-based coaching and conventional education
   b. Dependent variables include: attitudinal barriers, pain intensity, pain relief, functional status, and quality of life

4. Difficulty in keeping coaching intervention focused on pain, difficulty with attention-control phone calls turning into clinical support calls, high attrition due to death or disease progression, and more attrition in the coaching group.

Activity 3

1.

	Pretest	Teaching	Posttest
Group A	X	X	X
Group B		X	X
Group C	X		X
Group D			X

Note: The groups may be arranged in any order, but the four-group pattern must be followed.

2. The nurses would be randomly assigned to each of the groups using a table of random numbers or computer random assignment.
3. The pain knowledge and attitudes questionnaire would be used as a pretest.
4. The teaching program is the experimental treatment.
5. The pain knowledge and attitudes questionnaire is also the posttest or outcome measure.
6. The Solomon four-group design is ideal for experimental studies in which the pretest might affect the outcome. In this case, the questionnaire might change nurses' knowledge and attitudes about pain management. The researcher will be able to compare results for nurses receiving the teaching and not receiving the teaching with and without the pretest.

7. This type of design is particularly effective in ruling out threats to internal validity that the before-and-after groups may experience. It is effective for highly sensitive issues, which might be affected by simply completing a questionnaire as a baseline pretest.
8. A disadvantage of the Solomon four-group design is that a large number of subjects must be available for assignment into the four groups.

Activity 4

1. Quasi-experimental designs may be more practical, more feasible, and more adaptable to real-world practice. In many studies important to nursing, it is not possible to randomize subjects into groups for practical or ethical reasons.

2. The researcher must carefully examine other factors that could account for differences between groups.
3. The clinician must carefully critique the research study and also look for other factors, which might explain the results of the study. The results of any study with any design must be evaluated to determine if other factors influence the findings. The results should also be compared with the findings of other similar studies.

Activity 5: Web-Based Activity

1. This number will vary depending on when the search is conducted.
2. The types of articles will vary depending on when the search is conducted, but often you will find editorials, review articles, and research studies.
3. This number will vary depending on when the search is conducted.
4. This number will vary depending on when the search is conducted.

Activity 6: Evidence-Based Practice Activity

1. Level V
2. Level I
3. Level VI
4. Level II
5. Level III

POSTTEST

1. a. E
   b. Q
   c. E
   d. E
   e. Q
2. a. 3
   b. 1
   c. 2
   d. 6
   e. 4
   f. 5

CHAPTER 10

Activity 1

L O N G I T U D I N A L D M E
C I S P U E Q W H X O I Y H X
C R F L G Y Q E R C X E C G P
U W O L Z S B Q F H V O H H O
N T L S C I S Z A R R O I U S
L G T R S D L D U R Z L D O T
U E I O I S Q S E D L V W O F
I U W S J J E L O S Y U H I A
G T D K X O A C I E M D I I C
Q W R E E T O K T T E S T A T
A S A M I K E N B I B H U L O
D U O O K L H N P H O B Z V F
M C N G U L U E O L Y N R K C
K A M F G U P Q S B Z L A H T
L W J F V N E W J S W L E L V

1. Survey
2. Longitudinal
3. Correlational
4. Ex post facto
5. Cross-sectional
6. Correlational
7. Longitudinal
8. Survey
9. Cross-sectional
10. Comparative

Activity 2

	Advantages	Disadvantages
Correlation studies	A3	D1, D3, D4, D7
Cross-sectional	A1, A8	D2, D5
Ex post facto	A4	D1, D2, D3, D4, D5, D7
Longitudinal	A2, A6	D2, D8, D9
Prospective	A2, A7	D3, D4, D7, D8
Retrospective	A4	D1, D2, D3, D4, D5, D7
Survey	A1	D5, D7

Activity 3
1. ES: Exploratory survey
2. L: Longitudinal, or P: prospective
3. CS: Cross-sectional
4. R: Retrospective, or E: Ex post facto
5. C: Correlational
6. M: Methodological
7. MA: Meta-analysis

Activity 4
1. Longitudinal, descriptive
2. Yes:
   - Higher MFA will be negatively related to adverse neonatal outcomes.
   - Higher MFA will be positively related to improved health practices during pregnancy.
   - Improved health practices during pregnancy will be negatively related to adverse neonatal outcomes.
   - Health practices during pregnancy will mediate the relationship between MFA and adverse neonatal outcomes.
3. Inclusion criteria: participants had to be 16 years or older, between 24 and 28 weeks gestation with singleton pregnancies, and able to speak English.
   Exclusion criteria: prior to data collection they had been treated with tocolytic therapy, diagnosed with preeclampsia or gestational diabetes, diagnosed with a chronic medical condition (e.g., chronic hypertension, diabetes mellitus), or had an abnormal diagnostic result (e.g., known fetal anomaly, abnormal results on first or second trimester screening tests) during the current pregnancy. Additionally, women reporting a history of fetal (spontaneous abortion after 24 weeks gestation) or infant death were excluded. The inclusion criteria and the timing during pregnancy were chosen to try to increase the chances of MFA as the pregnancy progresses and MFA should increase. The exclusion criteria were chosen because of their known effect on neonatal outcomes. The aims of the study would be harder to demonstrate if the exclusion criteria were not used and they confounded the data.
4. Data were collected from the participants at one point during weeks 24-28 of their pregnancy. Additional data were collected from the medical record during this period and also within 48 hours of delivery.

Activity 5
Ex post facto design

Activity 6: Web-Based Activity
1. Answers for this activity will vary depending on when the search is conducted.
2. Answers for this activity will vary depending on when the search is conducted.

Activity 7: Evidence-Based Practice Activity
1. d
2. b
3. a, b

POSTTEST
1. Variables
2. Survey
3. Descriptive, exploratory, comparative
4. Relationship-difference

5. Correlational
6. Interrelational
7. Retrospective
8. a. Cross-sectional
   b. Longitudinal/prospective
   c. Retrospective/ex post facto
9. Cross-sectional; longitudinal
10. Prospective
11. Retrospective
12. Methodological

CHAPTER 11

Activity 1
1. Meta-analysis, systematic review
2. Integrative review
3. Meta-analysis
4. Clinical practice guidelines
5. Expert-based guidelines, evidence-based guidelines

Activity 2
1. In a good systematic review, the aims are clearly stated as a PICO statement and the eligibility and relevance criteria are well described and are predetermined. The reader can clearly see how the search relates to the aims and how studies included in the review fit eligibility criteria.
2. Transparency and reproducibility are important to convey in the methods section. The reader should feel confident that based on the article, they could recreate the literature search, data extraction, bias assessment, data combination, and quality appraisal and reach the same conclusions as the authors. The authors should also fully describe their inclusion and exclusion criteria and the rationale behind them.
3. The authors fully describe their search strategy, we look for evidence that they combed through all relevant databases and used their sources to search for literature in literature cited sections, bibliographies, etc. A good description of a rigorous search will leave the reader assured that all eligible studies have been located.
4. A good systematic review will document how the authors determined validity and reliability of the studies in the review (did they use a quality appraisal system? If so, which one?).

The authors will provide their grading scheme for determination of quality in the included studies. The reader will understand how the authors appraised the literature and how this appraisal led to the author's conclusions in the paper. The experience and qualifications of all reviewers should also be briefly described.
5. The authors provide the reader with a way to identify the studies used in the review and their findings and quality. Often, this is done in a table format. A good-quality table will allow the reader to understand the findings and will often lead naturally to a discussion where the author can easily synthesize the findings of the included studies.

Activity 3
1. SR, MA, IR
2. SR, IR
3. MA
4. IR
5. ECG, EBCG
6. EBCG
7. MA
8. ECG
9. ECG, EBCG
10. IR
11. MA

Activity 4
1. It is an expert-based clinical guideline. The guideline was based on a panel of national experts in child abuse. The policy provides guidelines for doctors, but does not provide an evidence table upon which the practice guideline was based.
2. Pediatricians
3. "The American Academy of Pediatrics recommends that pediatricians develop skills in the recognition of signs and symptoms of abusive head injury, including those caused by both shaking and blunt impact, consult with pediatric subspecialists when necessary, and embrace a less mechanistic term, abusive head trauma, when describing an inflicted injury to the head and its contents.

   "The goal of this policy statement is not to detract from shaking as a mechanism of AHT but to broaden the terminology to account for the multitude of primary and secondary injuries that result from AHT, some of which contribute to the often-permanent and significant brain damage sustained by abused infants and children."

4. The guideline provides pediatricians with 5 recommendations for practice including: learning the signs and symptoms, steps to providing a thorough assessment, subspecialist consultants who may be helpful, correct terminology for diagnosis and communication, and prevention efforts.

Activity 5

1. Systematic reviews can provide evidence for developing practice; reviews based on multiple RCTs provide stronger evidence. A meta-analysis can provide Level I evidence, the higher level of evidence. Systematic reviews can help clinicians to manage the expanding volume of research literature. The systematic review process and critiquing process help clinicians understand how to rate and use the information gleaned from multiple studies.

2. Clinical expertise and patient values or preference

3. b and d

4.

Level of Evidence	Description	Source
Level I	Meta-analysis of RCTs	C
Level II	A well-designed RCT	C
Level III	Quasi-experimental study	C
Level IV	Single nonexperimental study	C
Level V	Systematic review of qualitative studies	B, C
Level VI	Single descriptive or qualitative study	A
Level VII	Opinion of authorities, report of expert committee	A, E

POSTTEST

1. Integrative review
2. Quantitative
3. Systematic review and meta-analysis, meta-analysis
4. More than 1 person, excluded
5. Meta-analysis, highest level of evidence
6. Analysis
7. Bias
8. Forest plot, blobbogram
9. Evidence-based practice, expert-based guidelines
10. Does not, published studies

CHAPTER 12

Activity 1

1. Sample: Set of units that are selected to represent an entire population.
   Population: Well-defined set that has certain specified properties, may be defined broadly or narrowly.
   Differences: The population is the entire set of units with specified characteristics. The entire population is not often feasible to include in a study. The sample is a subset of the population that is selected to represent the entire population.

2. Target population: The entire population that meets the sampling criteria.
   Accessible population: A population that meets the target population criteria and that is available to the researcher.
   Differences: The target population is the whole, whereas the accessible population is the slice that is available to the researcher.

3. Inclusion criteria: Population descriptors used to select a sample.
   Exclusion criteria: Characteristics that restrict the population to make it more homogeneous.
   Differences: These terms describe the same concept. Inclusion, exclusion, eligibility, and delimitations are all terms used to describe subject attributes that researchers consider

when determining if the individual is part of a population.

Activity 2

1. Probability sampling uses random selection and is more rigorous. Nonprobability sampling uses nonrandom methods and there is no way to ensure that each element has a chance for inclusion in the sample.
2. a. N
   b. N
   c. P
   d. N
   e. P
   f. P

Activity 3

1. b
2. d
3. a
4. c
5. d
6. e
7. d

Activity 4

1. a. Yes, the sample is adequately described. The inclusion criteria were noted as (a) one or both members of the couple had been deployed to OIF or OEF while serving in the US Army, (b) both members could read and speak English, and (c) both members had been in a self-defined "committed relationship" for at least 1 year. In addition, both members of the couple had to be willing to consent to participate in the study.
   b. No, there were no statistically significant differences.
   c. Convenience
   d. Nonprobability
   e. The sampling unit was the couple.
   f. Packets were mailed to 85 couples, 66 couples returned completed surveys (77.6% response rate). Surveys were returned by couples in which the male was the service member (n = 39) and in which both members of the couple were in the military (n = 27). Seven packets were returned by only one member of the couple and therefore were not included. To more fully explore differences between

types of service, we compared active duty (n = 38 individuals), National Guard or reserve (n = 18 individuals), and soldiers who had left the Army and returned to civilian life after their most recent deployment (n = 35 individuals).
2. Subjects were accessible to the researcher, the researcher was able to assemble a sample meeting the inclusion criteria, and was able to get preliminary data on the role of resilience in military families.
3. Greater risk of bias, voluntary participation may skew results, less generalizability than other sampling methods
4. The researchers used multiple methods to recruit subjects (Facebook, veteran service organization blogs, veteran-targeted publications, fliers at military treatment facilities). These methods may help other researchers reach this population for future studies.

Activity 5

1. True
2. True
3. False
4. False
5. True
6. True
7. False

Activity 6

1. Yes, the characteristics of the sample were well described.
2. Adults with cancer-related pain receiving care at outpatient clinics.
3. The sample included mostly patients with lung, prostate, and head and neck cancers.
4. No. The sample contained 90% men in the control group, 95% in the education group, and 84% in the coaching group.
5. Yes. The criteria were: able to read and understand English, access to a telephone, a life expectancy longer than 6 months, average pain intensity score of 2 or higher as measured on a 0-10 scale, with higher scores meaning more pain.
6. Based on the material provided in the article, you could answer yes. The delimitation or exclusion criteria specified participants who had a concurrent cognitive or psychiatric condition or substance abuse problem that

would prevent adherence to the protocol, severe pain unrelated to their cancer, or resided in a setting where the patient could not self-administer pain medication.

7. The convenience sample was obtained by recruiting patients from six outpatient oncology clinics (three Veterans Affairs [VA] facilities, one county hospital, one community-based practice in California, and one VA clinic in New Jersey).

8. A convenience sample introduces more bias than any other sampling method; samples may not be representative of the population.

9. The sample size appears appropriate for this study. The authors state "To test the interaction of time (change in scores from pre- to post-study) by assignment to the three treatment groups (i.e., control, education, or coaching), a sample size of 240 was needed to detect a medium effect (f = 0.25; h2 = 6% of explained variance)." The authors had completed surveys from 289 participants after randomization to groups.

10. Yes, the study was approved by the institutional review board and research committee at each of the study sites.

Activity 7: Web-Based Activity

1. Answer will depend on state chosen and census year.

2. Answer will depend on state chosen and census year

3. "White. A person having origins in any of the original peoples of Europe, the Middle East, or North Africa. It includes people who indicate their race as "White" or report entries such as Irish, German, Italian, Lebanese, Arab, Moroccan, or Caucasian."

    "Black or African American. A person having origins in any of the Black racial groups of Africa. It includes people who indicate their race as "Black, African Am., or Negro"; or report entries such as African American, Kenyan, Nigerian, or Haitian."

4. The sample was 3.8% Black, 90.1% white. Comparisons between Table 1 in the study and census data will depend on the state chosen and the year of the census data.

Activity 8: Evidence-Based Practice Activity

The sample and sampling strategy is one variable that will influence the strength of the evidence provided by the study. The evidence from a meta-analysis of all *randomized* controlled trials is more influential in making practice change decisions than from a single descriptive or qualitative study with a convenience sample.

POSTTEST

1. Power analysis
2. Probability; nonprobability
3. Convenience
4. Simple random
5. Table of random numbers
6. Stratified random
7. Inclusion, exclusion criteria
8. Convenience, quota, purposive
9. Multistage or cluster
10. Data saturation

CHAPTER 13

Activity 1

1. Nursing research committee
2. Institutional review board
3. Justice
4. Expedited review
5. Unethical research study
6. HIPAA

Activity 2

1. Beneficence
2. Justice
3. Respect for person

Activity 3

Elements of Informed Consent

1. √ Title of protocol
2. √ Invitation to participate
3. 0 Basis for subject selection
4. √ Overall purpose of the study
5. √ Explanation of benefits
6. √ Description of risks and discomforts
7. √ Potential benefits
8. 0 Alternatives to participation

9. √   Financial obligations
10. √   Assurance of confidentiality
11. 0   In case of injury compensation
12. 0   HIPAA disclosure
13. √   Subject withdrawal
14. √   Offer to answer questions
15. √   Concluding consent statement
16. √   Identification of investigators

Activity 4
1. The elderly
2. Children
3. Pregnant women
4. The unborn

Other correct responses include those who are emotionally or physically disabled, prisoners, the deceased, students, and people with AIDS; also potentially includes oversubscribed research populations (organ transplantation patients, AIDS patients, "captive" and convenient populations).

Activity 5
1. a, c, d, f, g
2. a, b, c, d, f, g (Also, presume "e" was not adhered to because the study began in 1932 before IRBs and formal consent were required.)

Activity 6
1. Appendix A, Thomas et al., in the "Sample and Settings" section under "Methods," write, "The study was approved by the institutional review board and research committee at each of the sites." Under "procedures", write, "Prior to beginning participant recruitment, all research team members were trained extensively so that the procedures for enrollment, data collection, and interventions were standardized across all clinic sites. Research associates (RNs or psychology interns) were trained in procedures for evaluating potential participants, approaching them, obtaining consent to participate, and administering the instruments and videotapes. Patients were identified by clinic staff and screened for eligibility by the research associate, who then approached eligible patients, explained the study, and obtained written informed consent…. Participants received a $25 gift certificate after completing each set of questionnaires."

2. Appendix B, Alhusen et al., document in the "Data Collection Procedures" section of the article that "Institutional Review Board approval was obtained prior to participant recruitment. Eligible participants were approached about enrollment in the study during their prenatal care visits. If a woman expressed an interest in participating, but had not reached 24 weeks gestation, her contact information was obtained. The first author recontacted her and met with her to complete study instruments prior to a scheduled appointment that occurred between 24 and 28 weeks gestation. After a complete description of the study, informed consent was obtained from those women who agreed to participate. Participants were interviewed in a private space at each of the three study clinic sites. Interviews lasted approximately 30 minutes. The interviews were conducted by the first author or one of two undergraduate nursing students who received research compliance and study procedures training. Participants were compensated $15 for their participation."

3. Appendix C, Seiler et al., report in the "Data Collection Instruments" section, "Approval from a university Institutional Review Board was obtained prior to data collection. Each participant received an information letter that fully described the study, including the contact information of the researcher, a reminder that they could choose not to participate at any time and that they would be able to obtain the results of the study if interested. Informed consent was obtained from each participant to complete the demographic questionnaire and to audio record the interview. All identifying data were kept confidential in a locked file and were not included in the research report. No harm resulted from participating in the interview process. The participants benefited by sharing their first-hand experiences of providing health care to the homeless and aiding the interviewer and others to gain an understanding of their role."

4. Appendix D, Melvin et al., provide the least detailed description of how they protected human rights. They state in the "Participants" section under "Methods" that "Both members of the couple had to be willing to consent to participate in the study."

Under the "Procedures" section, they state "Demographic data were collected at the initial contact with one or both spouses, and included self-reported age, gender, military status (e.g., active duty, reserves), military rank (if applicable), race, ethnic status, current relationship status and duration, total number of marriages, number of children, and educational level. Study recruitment method also was documented (e.g., Facebook, newspaper, snowball)."

Activity 7: Web-Based Activity

1. The National Center on Shaken Baby Syndrome
2. The center educates parents and professionals and conducts research to prevent shaking and abuse of infants in the United States.
3. Ethical challenges to research with this population are that infants are considered a vulnerable population, as are pregnant women—a potential group for research on education and interventions to prevent infant abuse. Additionally, if there were an allegation of child abuse, the accused person may be a target for research to understand infant abuse. Children and infants cannot give informed consent, thus research on this group must be in consultation with an IRB. If a researcher found evidence of child abuse, he or she would be legally required to report it. Research trials on the effects of shaking abuse would be unethical. There are also other legal and ethical questions surrounding this population.

Activity 8: Evidence-Based Practice Activity

You could check the *Federal Register* or other government documents or websites to determine if misconduct had occurred, or check the journal for a correction or follow-up research report.

POSTTEST

1. Yes, because extra precautions should be taken to protect the rights of vulnerable populations, but this would not preclude undertaking research.
2. Before
3. Informed consent documents, IRB approval from the appropriate agency.
4. Yes

5. Informed consent
6. Risks to subjects may be greater than benefits, a patient's basic human rights could be violated, and results of a study would be questionable.

CHAPTER 14

Activity 1

Study 1 (Thomas et al.)

1. d
2. Six instruments were used: a demographic questionnaire, the Karnofsky Performance Status (KPS) scale, the Brief Pain Inventory (BPI), Barriers Questionnaire (BQ), Short Form Health Survey (SF-36), and the Functional Assessment of Cancer Therapy-General (FACT-G). The demographic questionnaire allowed researchers to collect age, education level, gender, ethnicity, marital status, living arrangements, and employment. The KPS measures functional status on a scale from 0-100 where higher scores indicate higher function, the BPI is a self-report instrument to measure the intensity and quality of pain. The BQ measures 8 attitudinal barriers to cancer pain management. The SF-36 measures functional status across 8 domains. The FACT-G measures quality of life. Questionnaires allow self-report data to be collected; measuring quality of life could not be accomplished through physiological instruments. Questionnaires are particularly useful for collecting data on experiences, feelings, behaviors, or attitudes. The authors did not find statistically significant changes in the scales over the course of the intervention; one possible reason they listed was that these measures were not sensitive enough to capture the changes following the intervention.

Study 2 (Alhusen et al.)

1. c/d/e
2. The participants were interviewed for about 30 minutes by the author or a nursing student and during that time they completed the three instruments: the Maternal-Fetal Attachment Scale (MFAS), the Health Practices in Pregnancy Questionnaire-II (HPQ-II), and a demographic and pregnancy measure. Additionally, neonatal outcomes

and maternal physical health risk factors were extracted from the medical record. Maternal-fetal attachment and health practices are an experience, feeling, behavior, or attitude and a questionnaire is the appropriate method for collecting this data. The medical record contains the record of neonatal outcomes and maternal physical health risk factors and is the appropriate place to collect this type of data. The rationale for use of an interview in this study was not described by the authors and the participants may have been able to complete the study instruments without the interview.

Study 3 (Seiler et al.)

1. c/d
2. The researchers wanted to understand the experiences of nurse practitioners who provide health care to the homeless. Interviews were audiotaped and used open-ended questions to learn about the experiences of nine nurse practitioners. There is a gap in knowledge of the experiences of advanced-practice nurses in caring for the homeless, since this study is building a knowledge base where there has not been previous research, the use of an interview is appropriate, and the use of a phenomenology lens allows the researchers to explore, analyze, and describe this experience. The authors also used a short demographic questionnaire to collect data on gender, race, marital status, family income, and NP position status. The interview method provides the most flexibility when used with open-ended questions to learn about the experience of caring for the homeless. One weakness of using a small sample such as this is that it lacks generalizability and may not be representative of the experience of all NPs who care for the homeless.

Study 4 (Melvin et al.)

1. d
2. The surveys used included: the Post-Traumatic Stress Symptoms Checklist (PCL),

the Revised Connor-Davidson Resilience Scale (R-CD-RISC), the Revised Dyadic Adjustment Scale (RDAS), the adapted gender-neutral Women's Experience of Battery (WEB), the Traumatic Experience Questionnaire (TEQ), and a demographic data measure that included age, gender, military status, military rank, race, ethnic status, current relationship status and duration, total number of marriages, number of children, and educational level, dates of deployment, location, and job while deployed.

3. The researchers kept the order of study survey measures constant to ensure that participants answered questions about their lifetime history of trauma prior to answering questions about PTSD. Both members of a couple had to agree to participate in the study. Surveys were mailed to both members of a couple in separate envelopes, and the participants were reminded that questions should be answered independently and that answers should not be discussed prior to returning the surveys. Although the researchers measured coercion and interpersonal violence, the study did not provide an avenue for researchers to report violence to clinicians or others in contact with the participants. The authors suggest that screening for violence in clinical settings should occur to protect both members of these military couples.

Activity 2

1. Consumers
2. Physiological
3. Reactivity
4. Interviews
5. Records
6. Questionnaire
7. Objectivity, consistency
8. Concealment
9. Interrater reliability
10. Operationalization
11. Likert scale
12. Content analysis
13. Fun

```
D E L I V E R S T A T I S T C S Y E S P A S
S S A C A B I N E T F O R K A Z O S P E I O
I A W O P E R A T I O N A L I Z A T I O N B
G T S N O R N E V E R B Y D N E A U X B T J
N S Y S T E M A T I C A J H T B S D V S E E
I F L I K E R T S C A L E E R R O Y A E R C
F A K S C A L E S N O V N O C A A U L R R T
H C U T A C R A T I M A P V E T P U I V A I
Y T B E B H I R T E M A H V W K I C D A T V
P C O N T E N T A N A L Y S I S P V O T E I
R O Y C B K D S I S R T S A D V A N E I R T
E R E Y O D U G K A T P I B I O I O G O R Y
A V S I B R Q U E S T I O N N A I R E N E C
C I A R E S E A R C H L L R E A C E S O L O
T O B M E X C E L A E O O D A T A C O V I N
I U E A E V A L I D S T G N O S T O O E A S
V N Y E S S I N T E R V I E W S A R F R B U
I H A P P I E N E S S P C A T A G D U N I M
T X C I T E D E L P H I A T O T P S N V L E
Y C E A T U B B S A N D L D O N N M A R I R
Y A B L E A C O N C E A L M E N T O O T T S
A I K E V A L I K E I I A B C O N S U M Y S
```

Activity 3

1. Children; interactions between people where the investigator is not part of the interaction; psychiatric patients; classrooms
2. The consent is usually of the type where permission to observe for a specified purpose is requested. The specific behaviors that are to be observed are not named. The use of the data and degree of anonymity are explained. In some situations, the subjects will be asked to review the data after the observation and before inclusion in the data pool.
3. Reactivity is the major concern, when the investigator has reason to believe that his or her presence will change the nature of the subjects' behavior.

Activity 4

Physiological measures would be of minimal use since the data being sought would not involve actual measures of the residents' physiological status. Not particularly interested in current blood pressure, temperature, urinary output, etc.

Could consider using observation; for example, sitting in an emergency department and observing the types of health care concerns that enter. Would need to think about whether this would be observation with concealment. Would need to wrestle with the notion of what is private information and what is public domain information. Also, would an emergency department provide information about all of the residents of the community and their health needs?

Could use questionnaires and collect data from all types of health care providers. Could provide a lot of data in a short time. Wonder how busy they would be and what would be the probability of their filling out the questionnaire? Do health providers have an idea of the health beliefs and practices of all of their patients?

Could use an interview. Is costly in terms of researcher time, but could provide more detailed information because subjects could be asked to expand on specific items. But who should be interviewed? How does one get into their offices/ homes, etc.?

Need to get some information from the people who actually live here. How could you reach a cross-section of the residents of your rural community? Could they be called? What about those people without a telephone?

Better check out the census data to get a clearer picture of what is being dealt with. Probably have some morbidity and mortality data collected by the state health department. Would probably use existing records to get a first sense of what the parameters of "health" are in this community. Then talk to some people about who knew the most about this area and arrange some interviews with these individuals. These would be guided interviews with open-ended items to encourage the sharing of as much information as possible. Would also seek a way to collect data from a variety of health care users; for example, surveys in the waiting room of various agencies, maybe the crowd at a mall, at a county fair.

One data collection instrument would not be sufficient to collect the information needed about the areas addressed.

Activity 5
1. d
2. a
3. d
4. a, b, c
5. d

Activity 6: Web-Based Activity
Answers will vary depending on when the search is conducted and what database is used.

Activity 7: Evidence-Based Practice Activity
Answers will vary depending on the topic chosen, when the search is conducted, and what database is used.

POSTTEST
1. d
2. d
3. c
4. b
5. b
6. d
7. c
8. d
9. b
10. b
11. b
12. d
13. a
14. d
15. a

CHAPTER 15

Activity 1
1. S; avoided by proper calibration of the scale.
2. S; decrease error by providing instructions, ensuring confidentiality, or other means to allow students to freely express themselves.
3. R; lessen by training research assistants and using strict protocols or rulebooks to guide analysis.
4. R; decrease their anxiety by addressing their concerns, providing comfort measures, or other efforts that might decrease their anxiety. Anxiety may alter the test responses.

Activity 2
1. Construct validity
2. Face validity
3. Content validity
4. Content validity index
5. Construct validity or convergent validity
6. Convergent validity; contrasted groups; divergent validity; factor analysis; hypothesis testing
7. Contrasted groups

Activity 3
1. Stability; homogeneity; equivalence
2. Test-retest methods could be accomplished by giving the same test again at a later date and seeing if the two scores are highly correlated. Parallel or alternate forms, such as alternate versions of the same test, could also be used to establish stability.
3. Alternate forms would be better if the test-taker is likely to remember and be influenced by the items or the answers from the first test.
4. a. 2
   b. 4
   c. 1
   d. 3
5. a. A Likert scale is commonly used when measuring psychosocial variables or attitudes. It asks respondents to respond to a question using a scale of varying intensity between two extremes. We would expect the scale to ask if the respondent strongly agrees or disagrees with a statement or if the statement is "most like me or least like me" on a scale from 1-5 where one is anchored by being least like me.

b. Was developed to measure posttraumatic stress symptoms in military and civilian populations. Was reported to be valid based on correlations between the PCL and the clinician-administered PTSD scale.

c. The information provided for the instrument would increase confidence in the results of the study. Based on the descriptions, the instrument chosen was appropriate. If a greater understanding of the instruments is needed, the original articles referenced in this study would be a good place to start. Additional studies of the measures used could also provide information on recent changes or adaptations of the measures.

Activity 4
Results will depend on the search term chosen and availability of psychometric testing information on the chosen instrument.

Activity 5
1. Six instruments, the Karnofsky Performance Status (KPS) scale, the Brief Pain Inventory (BPI), The Barriers Questionnaire (BQ), the Short Form Health Survey (SF-36), the Functional Assessment of Cancer Therapy-General (FACT-G), and a demographic questionnaire developed for this study.

2. a. No specific information on validity was given, but the author states that reliability and validity are well-established and does give a reference.
   b. No
   c. Cronbach's alpha, test-retest reliability, item-total correlations and inter-item correlations for each domain in the scale, split-half, parallel or alternate form.
   d. No, it is used for yes/no format questionnaires; the FACT-G uses a 5-point Likert scale.
   e. Yes, the authors state that it has been used in patients with cancer and in patients with cancer-related pain.
   f. You would start with the reference given for reliability and validity and you may complete a search of reliability and validity on this instrument.
   g. You would read the discussion section; the authors do compare their results to

other studies and discuss the differences on subscale scores. This is also a good place to look for discussion about threats to internal or external validity.

Activity 6: Evidence-Based Practice Activity
First, this study would need to be put into context. It would need to be known what other studies were available in the same area. If a decision were being made based solely on the published reliability and validity information, it would not be considered a strong study.

To qualify this statement, there may be more information about the reliability and validity of the instruments. Some of it may have been cut to meet required article length. Some information is given, and what is presented is valuable and does lead to some confidence in the results—certainly more confidence than if they had been using several newly constructed instruments.

A final answer would be "it depends." Some questions would need to be asked and a deeper literature search on maternal-fetal attachment would need to be done.

POSTTEST
1. Cronbach's alpha
2. Concurrent
3. Convergent
4. Content
5. Factor analysis
6. Interrater
7. Test-retest
8. Content
9. Convergent
10. Cronbach's alpha

CHAPTER 16

Activity 1
You will have your set of completed cards.

Activity 2
1. d
2. c
3. d
4. a
5. a, b, or c, depending on the tool used to measure satisfaction
6. a

7. b
8. d
9. a
10. c
11. d

Activity 3

Across

1. j   Goofy's best friend
3. e   Old abbreviation for mean
5. b   Abbreviation for number of measures in a given data set (the measures may be individual people or some smaller piece of data such as blood pressure readings)
8. m   Describes a set of data with a standard deviation of 3 when compared with a set of data with a standard deviation of 12
10. h   Abbreviation for standard deviation
11. f   Marks the "score" where 50% of the scores are higher and 50% are lower
12. c   Measure of variation that shows the lowest and highest number in a data set

Down

1. l   The values that occur most frequently in a data set
2. i   68% of the values in a normal distribution fall between ±1 of this statistic
4. d   Can describe the height of a distribution
6. g   Describes a distribution characterized by a tail
7. k   Very unstable
9. a   Measure of central tendency used with interval of ratio data

Activity 4

1. a. adverse neonatal outcomes
    b. nominal dichotomous variable
2. a. Maternal-fetal attachment (MFA)
    b. adverse neonatal outcome
    c. In order to use inferential statistics, we know that it must be at interval or ratio level. The MFAS used a Likert scale and there is no stated absolute zero, so it must be interval level.
3. a. A dyad is two individuals who are regarded as a pair in the analysis. The authors used a dyad in their analysis since "Because both spouses completed separate surveys, yet they were describing the same marital relationship, this

interdependence can produce significant correlations in survey scores. Therefore our chosen analysis method accounted for interdependence of couple measures." (Melvin et al. 2012).
    b. Nominal or ordinal; is a test of the difference between groups

Activity 5

1. Null hypothesis
2. Parametric statistics
3. Research hypothesis
4. Sampling error
5. Parameter; statistic
6. Correlation
7. Type II error; Type I error
8. Probability
9. Practical significance
10. Nonparametric statistics
11. Statistical significance
12. Research hypothesis; null hypothesis
13. c, b, a, e, d

Activity 6

1. N = 12
2. Nominal, ordinal, interval
3. 7.6
4. 6
5. 3
6. Limited sample size, N = 12; every score affects the mean

Activity 7

1. a. Yes
    b. Yes
    c. Yes
    d. Yes
2. All studies used descriptive statistics to describe certain characteristics of the sample (e.g., age, sex, ethnicity, marital status, income).
    a. sample size (N), mean, standard deviation (SD), range
    b. N, mean, SD, range, median
    c. N, frequency, %
    d. N, %, mean, SD, Z score
3. a. Yes
    b. Yes
    c. Yes
    d. Yes
4. Yes, the Melvin et al. and Alhusen et al. studies were descriptive studies.

5. a. Yes
   b. Yes
   c. No
   d. Yes
6. a. Chi square ($\chi2$), ANCOVA
   b. Logistic regression, Pearson correlation, bivariate correlation, multiple regression
   c. None used because this is a qualitative study
   d. Multiple regression, t-test, chi square ($\chi2$)

Activity 8: Web-Based Activity

1. a. We can surmise that a wider confidence interval is an indication of more uncertainty in the estimate, since the population standard and standard deviations are estimated from the data. If there are limited data to estimate the standard deviation, we will expect a wider CI due to this uncertainty. We can feel more confident that if we were to sample the same population repeatedly, we would get a confidence interval that would bracket the true population standard in 95% of the cases.
   b. Percentages, incidences, median, range, average

Activity 9: Evidence-Based Practice Activity

The nurses should stop and consider how their actions could make a difference. They could check out the websites that are listed as references on the child abuse prevention site and look for recommendations of experts in the field. They could anticipate finding guidelines for ways of preventing abusive head trauma and could evaluate ways to include those recommendations in their practice. They could provide literature or education for parents both before the child is born and during infancy. They may also need to devise a way to collect data for an evaluation of the steps they had taken (such as by evaluating the effect of their educational materials, evaluation of how often they are providing education during clinic visits, etc.).

POSTTEST

1. This is a matter of personal preference and of probability. At clinic 1 you would have a longer average wait time, but 68% of the wait times would be from 30 to 50 minutes.

At clinic 2, you may have a shorter wait sometimes, but 68% of the wait times would be between 0 and 70 minutes.

2. The mean would provide information about the most common number of hospital gowns needed on your unit, but it is sensitive to outliers. The median could also be examined, but it is not clear if the hospital gown data has a normal distribution. Perhaps the best method would be to look at both the mean and median to determine the number of gowns for your unit. The mode may be useful, but again without knowing the distribution of the data, there is no way to know if the gown data has one mode or is bimodal. The mode would be less useful than the median and mean.

3. Mode------------ Most frequent score
   Median----------Middle score
   Mean -----------Arithmetical average – most stable

4. Nonsymmetrical, positive, negative
5. Hypothesis
6. Sampling distributions, inferential
7. Null hypothesis
8. Type II error
9. Chi-square

CHAPTER 17

Activity 1

1. R
2. D
3. R
4. D
5. R
6. R
7. D

Activity 2

1. d
2. b
3. a
4. e
5. c

Activity 3

1. T
2. F
3. F

4. T
5. T
6. F

POSTTEST

1. The researchers identified four hypotheses. They were that (1) couple functioning as perceived by each member of the couple would be negatively associated with PTSS in one or both members of the couple, (2) the relationship between couple functioning and PTSS would be increased in magnitude by lower level of resilience, younger age, female gender, lower military rank, increased levels of trauma exposure, and marital conflict resolution problems, (3) difference in perceptions of couple functioning between female or dual military soldier couples, and (4) that STS would be present in 12-70% of civilian spouses in the study sample. The results of each hypothesis are presented in the Results section.

2. Information regarding the results for each hypothesis is presented concisely. In addition the researchers present the information on each hypothesis sequentially, stating "the first hypothesis" and "second hypothesis" when presenting the results for the first two hypotheses. The last two hypotheses are presented sequentially, but not labeled as such.

3. The tests that were used to analyze the data are identified for the first hypothesis (general linear mixed model) and for the third hypothesis (Chi-square analysis).

4. Yes, the results are presented objectively. The researchers avoided opinions or reactionary statements about the data.

5. Table 1, Table 2, and Table 3 are used to supplement the presentation of the results. There is information (mostly data or numbers) that is only found in the tables. Only a minimal amount of information in the tables is repetitive of the text. This information was often the mention of a P value for the results in both the table and text. All of the tables have precise headings.

6. Although the results are interpreted in light of the hypotheses, the researchers do not apply the findings back to the theoretical framework that was chosen to guide the study.

7. Although the some of the hypotheses were supported (i.e., the second hypothesis was not supported), the researchers did not provide a discussion of how the theoretical framework was supported.

8. The researchers make several statements about the weakness of the study. For example, they discuss the low reliability of the Trauma Event Questionnaire and the cross-sectional study design. The also identified study strengths. For example, they found PTSS demonstrated a similar effect on couple functioning in both male and dual military couples who have deployed, which is a finding not previously reported.

9. The researchers discuss the study's clinical relevance throughout the discussion section. For example, they state that "the finding that couples with high resilience also had higher couple functioning despite high levels of PTSS provides a starting place for the development of preventative interventions." The researchers also indicate that "nurses and other healthcare professionals should also ensure accurate documentation of trauma history and referrals for treatment during interactions with military couples as indicated."

10. The researchers avoid making any grand generalizations. Much of the discussion is related to previous literature on similar topics. In addition, the researchers go so far as to state the reasons why they believe that "the complex nature of how couples are affected by combat-related PTS cannot be fully explained in the sample."

11. The researchers state recommendations for future research. For example, the researchers state that determining the direction of the relationship between coercion, interpersonal violence, and couple functioning is an "important goal for future research." In addition, the researchers also state that "the relationships in this study should be further explored using other methods, such as longitudinal data collected before and after deployment, to better evaluate causality patterns and the presence of mediators." Further recommendations are provided in the final paragraph of the study.

CHAPTER 18

Activity 2

Please note that what follows are the results of one inspectional reading of the study by Thomas et al. (2012). You are not expected to agree with these findings. Some of you may agree, but some of you may not.

Systematic skimming: In reading the title, abstract, the biographies, and the discussion, the following conclusions were made:

- The biographical information of the authors/researchers indicates that they have a clinical nursing background in oncology and research/statistical methods.
- The PICO of the scenario could be P: inpatient clients with cancer, I: interventions for pain management/control, C: usual care, O: pain. The PICO of the study is similar to the PICO from the scenario. The PICO from the study would be P: outpatient clients with cancer who have a life expectancy > 6 months and a pain intensity score > 2; I_1: video + educational, I_2: video + education + coaching; C: video; O: pain intensity, pain relief, pain interference, attitudinal barriers, functional status, quality of life.
- Yes, would proceed to superficial reading.

Superficial reading:
1. Remembered about the study:
   - Two interventions, one control group; an experimental study
   - Hypotheses
   - Convenience sample but allocation was stratified based on pain and cancer treatment
   - There was randomization, blinding
   - Reliable and valid data collection tools, references provided
   - This would be Level II evidence
   - The study was approved by an ethics board
   - Figures and tables with data
   - Data analysis section
   - Results section
   - Discussion section
   - Reread this study in greater detail and consider for critical appraisal. It continues to appear to be relevant to the scenario.

Activity 3

An experimental study of moderate to strong quality, given that the strengths outweigh the limitations, was conducted in a sample of primarily men, 60 years of age, who have been diagnosed with multiple types of cancer, and were seeking outpatient care. Participants were randomized to receive one of two interventions (education alone or education plus coaching) or usual care. The only significant differences between the groups were for pain interference scores and mental health component of the SF-3. Participants who received the education plus coaching intervention had a significantly lower pain interference scores and higher mental health scores at the end of the study (12 weeks) than those who received education alone or usual care. Based on the findings of this one study, a recommendation to not implement an education plus coaching intervention to improve pain management control practices among inpatient adult oncology patients could be determined.

CHAPTER 19

Activity 1

1. a. P—older adults
   b. I—adiposity, cardiorespiratory fitness
   c. C—none*
   d. O—mortality
   e. Prognosis
2. a. P—patients with diabetic foot ulcers
   b. I—negative pressure wound therapy (NPWT) using vacuum-assisted closure
   c. C—advanced moist wound therapy (AMWT)
   d. O—wound healing
   e. Therapy
3. a. P—adolescent clinical patients
   b. I—CRAFFT
   c. C—none*
   d. O—screening for substance abuse
   e. Diagnosis
4. a. P—children
   b. I—residential exposure to power line magnetic fields
   c. C—none*
   d. O—ALL
   e. Causation/Harm
*Note in some studies, there is no comparison

Activity 2

1. Therapy; Prognosis; Causation; Review; Qualitative
2. None
3. Clinical Trial; Meta-Analysis; Practice Guideline; Randomized Controlled Trial
4. Etiology; Diagnosis; Therapy; Prognosis; Clinical Predication Guides
5. PUBMED (Medline)—"Clinical Queries"

Activity 3

1. g
2. c
3. h
4. a
5. e
6. j
7. b
8. f
9. i
10. k
11. d

Activity 4

1. The percentage of patients who had bleeding; discrete/dichotomous.
2. "1.0." Note: The null value varies depending on the outcome; for a continuous outcome variable, the null value would be "0.0."
3. We are 95% certain that when a patient receives the pressure bandage they will be anywhere from 0.3 to 0.9 times less likely to experience bleeding than patients who did not receive the pressure bandage.
4. The risk of bleeding is 0.52 times less in patients who received pressure bandages than those who did not receive pressure bandages. The RR (or treatment effect) is statistically significant because the 95% Confidence Interval (0.3, 0.9) does not include 1.0 (the null value).
5. Thirty-two (32) patients need to be treated with pressure bandages in order to prevent bleeding in 1 patient. The NNT was calculated first by finding the absolute risk reduction (ARR), then dividing 1 by the ARR. The ARR = 6.7% − 3.4% = 3.2%. Then 1 is divided by 3.2% (or 1/0.032) = 31.25, which is rounded up to 32. Because pressure bandages are already being implemented in the scenario, there is research evidence to support the continued use to decrease bleeding. Implementation issues (i.e., cost, time, manpower) have likely already been addressed. However, the study also showed a significant increase in nausea and pain, so perhaps patient preferences may be considered in future discussions about implementation of pressure bandages.
6. Although there was a significant reduction in bleeding among patients who received the pressure bandages, there is likely research evidence to support the continued implementation of pressure bandages in the given scenario. However, in continuing the implementation, the RN should consider if (a) the population in the study is similar to his or her clinical situation (target population) and that (b) the application of results of the study to the target population should be done with caution, until higher level evidence (i.e., systematic review, practice guideline) is available.

Activity 5

1. P—U.S. teenage girls; I—not applicable; C—not applicable; O—eating disorders
2. There would be concern that the difference in geographic locations of the target population (California) and study population (Spain) would be significantly different even though the clinical situation PICO question and study question are similar.
3. Causation because the clinical situation and study are about determining whether one thing is related to another; based on the study design (cohort study) you would select the CASP Tool for Cohort Studies.
4. a. Discrete/dichotomous
   b. Discrete/dichotomous
   c. Discrete/dichotomous
   d. Discrete/dichotomous
5. Teenage girls whose parents were not married, who ate alone, who read girls' magazines more than once per week, and who listened to the radio for more than 1 hour per day were at increased odds for developing an eating disorder; all of these variables (except for "reading girls' magazines more than once per week") were statistically significantly associated with an increase in odds for developing an eating disorder; the null value is "1.0"; the CI for the variables of "parents' marital status", "eating alone", and "listening

to the radio" do not include "1.0," indicating that these results are statistically significant, whereas the CI for the "reading girls' magazines more than once per week" (0.91 to 2.2) includes "1.0," indicating that it is not statistically significant.

6. Although results of this study reflect a population of teenage girls from Spain, it is possible that there may be credibility in applying the evidence to the current clinical situation. Although an evidence-based practice change may not be warranted by this one study, a further review, critical appraisal, and synthesis of the evidence could lead to changes in screening teenage girls for eating disorders in the target population.

POSTTEST

1. False; an experimental or quasi-experimental study design is usually used for the therapy category of clinical concern used by clinicians; causation/harm studies typically use nonexperimental (longitudinal or retrospective) study designs.
2. True
3. True
4. False; sensitivity is the proportion of those with the disease who test positive and specificity is the proportion of those without the disease who test negative.
5. False; the CI provides the reader information about both the statistical and clinical significance of the findings. Although findings may be statistically significant, the clinician must apply the "low" and "high" end of the confidence levels to determine clinical significance.
6. True
7. True
8. False; likelihood ratio is a term used to describe the number that expresses the sensitivity, specificity, PPV, NPV, and prevalence for diagnosis clinical category questions.

CHAPTER 20

Activity 1

1. Evidence-based practice is a broader term that encompasses research utilization. Research utilization is focused on the application of research findings, whereas evidence-based practice is focused on the application of best-available evidence, which includes research findings in addition to nonresearch findings such as case reports and expert opinion.
2. a. the best-available evidence
   b. clinical expertise
   c. patient values

Activity 2

1. b
2. d
3. a
4. c
5. b
6. d

Activity 3

a. 4
b. 1
c. 5
d. 10
e. 2
f. 11
g. 7
h. 9
i. 3
j. 6
k. 8

Activity 4

1. Problem-focused; Knowledge-focused
2. Stakeholder(s)
3. Patient, Population, or Problem; Intervention/Treatment; Comparison Intervention/Treatment; Outcome(s)

Activity 5

1. Y
2. N
3. Y
4. N
5. N
6. Y

Activity 6

1. a. the nature of the innovation (e.g., the type and strength of evidence)
   b. the manner in which the innovation is communicated
2. a. 3
   b. 4

    c. 1

    d. 2

3. a. Y

    b. Y

    c. N

    d. Y

POSTTEST

1. Pediatric cardiology on 14 diagnosis groups
2. "Appointed CPG coordinator and the collaboration of all members of the healthcare team. The CPG steering group consists of expert clinicians, including the Vice President of Cardiovascular Critical Care Services, attending cardiologists, anesthesiologists and surgeons, clinical coordinators, nurse practitioners, staff nurses, patient care coordinator, respiratory therapists, nutritionist, and social worker" (Poppleton, Moynihan, & Hickey, 2003, p. 76).
3. It appears that all members of the team could be considered stakeholders; key stakeholders not represented could include patients (if applicable due to age), patients' families, senior hospital leadership (both medical and nursing).
4. Not indicated
5. Not indicated
6. Not indicated
7. Not indicated; not indicated
8. To a degree; however, recommendations are missing an indication to the evidence to support the recommendations and the grade of the evidence.
9. Not indicated
10. Detailed methodology for how patient data would be collected, including an excerpt from a sample clinical guideline and a variance-tracking sheet for a sample clinical guideline
11. Yes; yes, "the CPG Program has been a successful strategy in a continual effort to provide cost effective care without compromising quality" (Poppleton et al., 2003, p. 83), the authors report several positive outcomes
12. CPG coordinator could be considered both "Change Champion" (due to clinical expertise qualities) and "Opinion Leader" (due to technological qualities), both of which encompass EBP expertise; didactic education (education during orientation and when new CPGs are introduced)

CHAPTER 21

Activity 1 Your answers may vary.

	Quality Improvement	**Evidence-Based Practice**	**Research**
Purpose	Improve internal practices or processes	Change or reinforce nursing practice	Generate knowledge
Rigor ↔ Control	Protocols less formal/rigorous, may change throughout project	Interventions are more strict than QI, but not as controlled as research	Tight control of variables
Method	TQM/CQI Six Sigma Lean Clinical Microsystems	Iowa model of EBP Johanna Briggs institute model of EBP	Qualitative, quantitative, or mixed methods
Human subjects	Doesn't usually require IRB approval	Doesn't usually require IRB approval	Requires IRB approval unless exempt
Data collection	Benchmarking Collecting and monitoring data Rapid cycle	Literature search and appraisal Data collection not as rapid as QI	Observation, self-report, physiological, medical records, databases Data collection time varies
Results	Improve process	Treatments or nursing care are based on the best available evidence	Adds to the body of scientific knowledge
Dissemination	Within a unit or an agency	Publications, conferences, consultations, training programs, changing practitioner behavior through interaction with those who provide direct care	Scientific community, publications, conferences

Activity 2 Your answers may vary.
1. All use a systematic process.
2. The basic process is similar; all use systematic reasoning to address a clinical issue.
3. All provide evidence for quality care; QI provides the lowest strength and generalizability, while research provides the strongest evidence with the greatest generalizability.
4. Results of all three are disseminated, just on a different range.
5. All are collaborative processes.

Activity 3

You may fit the steps into the table differently, but be sure that all of the QI steps are included.

Quality Improvement	Nursing Process
1. Assess system performance by collecting/monitoring data. Data may include check or data sheets, surveys, interviews, or focus groups.	1. Assessment: collecting, organizing, and analyzing information or data about the patient. Subjective or objective data. Collected by observation, interview, examination. Data are reviewed and interpreted. Develop problem list and prioritize patient's problems.
2. Analyze data to ID problems in need of improvement. Determine if problem is due to common cause or special cause variation. Methods for analysis include: run charts, control charts, histograms, pie or bar charts, cause/effect diagrams, fishbone diagrams, RCA, tree diagram, 5 why's, flow chart.	2. Nursing diagnosis. Statement that describes and actual or potential problem.
3. Develop a plan for improvement. Develop and test a plan to treat the performance problem. May use the Model of Improvement.	3. Plan. Devise plan using patient goals and nursing orders to provide care that will meet patient's needs. Set patient goals.
4. Test and implement the plan. Use the PDSA cycle, use small and rapid tests of change. Evaluate success of the intervention, monitor system performance, track stability and sustainability of your change.	4. Implement. Carry out the nursing care plan you devised. Reassess the patient. Validate that the care plan is accurate. Implement nursing orders. Document.
5. Continue test and implement phase. Monitor system performance over time. Compare results to baseline.	5. Evaluate. Compare patient's current status with stated goals. Were goals achieved? Review nursing process.

Activity 4. Web-Based Activity

Suggestions for hospital improvement will vary based on survey results and individual experience.

Activity 5. Evidence-Based Practice Activity

Results will vary with topic chosen.

POSTTEST

1. Safe, effective, patient-centered, timely, efficient, equitable
2. Benchmarking
3. Assess system performance, analyze data to identify problems, develop a plan, test and implement the improvement plan
4. Support staff, patients, families
5. Common cause variation, special cause variation
6. SQUIRE
7. Plan, Do, Study, Act, Improvement Model

Notes

Notes

Notes

Notes